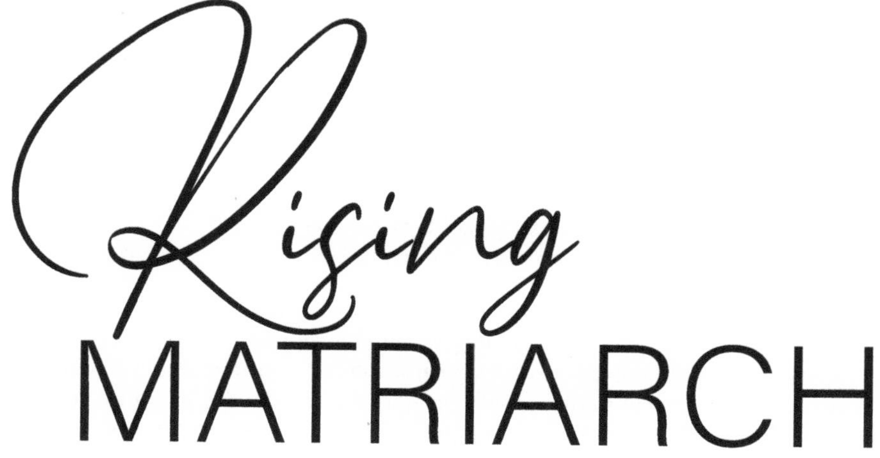

Rising MATRIARCH

STORIES OF WOMEN WHO REMEMBERED THEIR TRUTH & POWER

Beautiful Katie,
Thankyou for coming on my podcast,
I hope this book finds a special
place within your heart!

♡ Bee

First published in Australia in 2021
by KMD Books
Waikiki, WA 6169

Cover Design: Dylan Ingram
Interior Design: Chelsea Wilcox

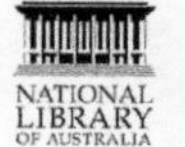

A catalogue record for this work is available from the National Library of Australia

National Library of Australia Catalogue-in-Publication data:
Rising Matriarch/Laura Elizabeth

ISBN: 978-0-6451353-5-0
(Paperback)

ISBN: 978-0-6451353-6-7
(eBook)

Foreword

In unity, we honour and pay our respects to the custodians of Whadjuk Noongar boodjar (country), the lands on which this book was first seeded.

We pay our respects to the Elders both past and present and to those emerging.

The stories woven within these pages may contain sensitive content and/or memories of loved ones who have passed on, which could activate a response within you.

Please read with awareness and care.

Welcome to the Rising Matriarch …

The deep dive to discover what it means to be a woman in her power.

What does she look like?

Dedicated to being of service to the rising feminine, and thus the healing of the collective consciousness, each woman's story woven within these pages offers a personal understanding and insight into what it means to embody a powerful woman.

May you hear our voices, may you witness our courage and may you feel inspired to ignite your own power within …

Contents

Introduction

Laura has a natural ability of bringing people together and building community. This book is no different and the inspiration for this project sang deeply into her bones.

Having just contributed to two other anthology books, Laura's yearning to keep writing was palpable. One afternoon as she stood barefoot looking out into the beauty of the bushland surrounding her, she received a breathtaking vision of women coming together to share their stories of healing, courage and empowerment that would inspire thousands of women around the globe.

Magic happens when women come together.

When we speak up and tell our stories, it gives others permission to do the same.

From there, this vision grew stronger and stronger. It became clear to Laura that this book was part of a deep calling to find these incredible women so that they can share their story's with the world.

She began to visualise and call in the energies of like-minded, powerful and inspiring women who were ready to step up and be seen. The result? An extremely diverse collective of amazing women, with incredibly inspiring stories to share.

This process, like any writing journey, has left no stone unturned for these authors. They heard the call to be seen and heard like never before, They have committed to being a leader and way shower for those feeling alone, stuck or lost.

This book will take you on a path of self discovery, push the limits of your comfort zone and inspire you to keep digging for the truth of who you are; a powerful Rising Matriarch.

Flavours & Magic

Laura Elizabeth

There are no obvious physical attributes to a woman who stands willingly in her power.

You cannot tell by her appearance, the etches and scars on her body, or the colour of her skin. You cannot tell by the clothes she wears, or the size of her smile.

When a woman is in her power, she simply … just is!

She feels the depths of her truth pumping at lightspeed through her veins. She embodies all of the wisdom of her ancestors within each and every cell of her body, like a badge of honour. She requires no validation, nor does she owe you an explanation.

There is no need for you to see or feel it. Only *she* decides how to reclaim her flavour of magic, woven through time and space.

She is no longer striving to become or emerge as a preconceived idea for you to be comfortable with, for she fully accepts herself and is consciously being.

Since the tender age of 16, I have dedicated my life to exploring and deepening an understanding of spiritual processes. This has translated into a developing career as a spiritual guide, leading clients back into discovering the truth of who they are at their core, using a variety of tools and modalities.

In the last few years, I have been compelled to follow a deeper path that focuses this guidance towards women. In particular, guiding their journey of unravelling limiting beliefs and conditioned behaviours, traumas and past life baggage, into a renewed place of embodying unique and innate wisdom, through the process of harnessing their erotic power and essence.

By remembering the sacredness of our intuition and sensuality and reconnecting to natural cycles, we can embrace our bodies and deepen connection to our yoni (vulva/vagina) and tapestry of collective womb consciousness.

Devoting my life's work to honouring women in this way is an absolute privilege beyond comprehension and words.

This sacred women's work grants me daily access to exploring the magnitude of experiences and potential power that can manifest within the vastness of a woman's flesh.

Every time I step into this space, I witness a rebirth. An awakening. A reclamation of ownership and acceptance.

Every day, I am given the opportunity to see nothing but beauty, compassion and magnificence in each client drawn to walk this path to truth with me. And thus, an invitation for me to gaze into those reflections and choose compassion, embodiment and acceptance of myself.

There is no doubt about it. Magic happens when women work together.

It can be gentle, or fierce. It can be both. I can be both, as can you!

The embodiment of this energy dances upon our skin, flows through our hair and bleeds from our womb. It is tangible, and once you taste a sip from that Holy Grail on your lips, you are hooked on a journey into self love.

What would change in your world right now, if you chose to lovingly and supportively accept all facets of self?

All of my experience thus far, has emphasised that the process of locating and harnessing that inner power is less likely to be a gentle and passive conscious choice, but a journey of collecting and enduring stories, that twist, shape, mould and test our very fibres.

Is your chosen fabric strong enough to weave a journey that will weather all seasons?

Take for instance my personal narrative of unraveling years (*lifetimes*) of bullshit and conditioned beliefs to keep me small, scared and afraid of my own voice …

I cultivated an outpouring of painful experiences one. After. The. Other. To fulfill an inherited doctrine that women should be seen and not heard. I was bullied all through high school. Filled with hatred for my body Told that I was disgusting … gross … ugly because of my rapid changing adolescent form and my textbook acne encrusted skin. I was catcalled, groped and intimidated by men every day from the age of twelve … TWELVE!

At the same time, I was also bullied by a family friend, to the point I would have panic attacks before a gathering, because this woman (old enough to be my mother, and certainly old enough to know better), had three daughters, one the same age as me, which somehow gave her the authority to terrorise and humiliate me for several years. Until finally, one day, my Mother cut ties and we no longer had to see that family. Was this woman jealous of a 12 year old? Who the fuck even knows? As far as I'm concerned there is no excuse for that kind of behaviour between an adult and child, but it happened … and it fit neatly into the suitcase of fear, shame and self loathing that followed every timid breath I took.

As a teenager, I wanted to disappear. I found comfort in music and pretending I was someone else.

There were times I wanted to die.

Those impressionable years cemented solid foundations of a *people pleasing* nature. I avoided conflict, instead trying to fly under the radar, and all forms of public speaking. I relinquished my voice simply to keep the peace.

I was brought up with a great sense of humour and coupled it with a grandiose alter ego to mask pain and loneliness.

For the record, I'm still hilarious. I enjoy laughter to *break state* and create a sense of safety for others around me, rather than a self-soothing or avoidance technique. (However, there would be some of my nearest and dearest who'd call bullshit on that being entirely true, one hundred percent of the time, ha!)

So I lived this way, relatively numb to emotion...

Back story; Growing up in a small fishing village on the North East Coast of central Scotland, I was shown from an early age that having, displaying and processing emotions was a sign of weakness, and needed to be controlled or suppressed, or I'd be ridiculed.

As such, I don't have strong memories of outwardly showing or receiving affection and words of affirmation as a child.

It wasn't the done thing.

I do feel overall, I experienced a joyful childhood within my family home. It just wasn't a heart-on-your-sleeve vibe.

Just for a laugh, I want to ask you right now, if you can guess what you feel my two main love languages might be?

Yep! Physical touch and words of affirmation!

And because the universe also has a strong sense of humour, what do I spend ninety percent of my time facilitating for my clients? Emotional breakthroughs!

You can't make this shit up. Our biggest fears and greatest challenges are truly our greatest breakthroughs and triumphs.

… Back to living this way, relatively numb to emotion and detached from truth. I was stuck in a cycle of existing for many years without even realising.

Fast forward to becoming a mother for the first, second and third time, and the feelings could no longer be ignored.

The birth of my children and the process of adapting to motherhood forced me to open Pandora's box of emotions, and allow myself to feel the ultimate unconditional love and expansion from places I never knew existed. But it meant finally addressing the malevolent threads of self-loathing that were pushed down for all those years.

Conveniently slapped with a post-natal depression and anxiety label, to make those around me feel more comfortable with my unravelling, I knew it went deeper than that. I knew I had vast layers of wounding, shame and toxic beliefs piled on top of each other that needed to be acknowledged, felt, released, healed and forgiven.

Now that I was responsible for three other lives, this journey of remembering and honouring my truth had become urgent and no longer negotiable. What example would I be leading if I didn't?

Squeezed perilously through the eye of an unforgiving needle. I was forced to face the darkest of demons. I was forced to face myself, all the while, clinging on to the hope and unconditional love held in the gazes of my children. If they believed in me, that was enough motivation to begin to love and save myself. To be my own superhero.

"Own your shit!"

And that's exactly what I did. I became consciously aware of who I was and what I was feeling. I acknowledged both the light and darkness in my behaviours, choices and mindset. It was a bitter pill to swallow at times, (even now!)

This newfound realness pissed a lot of people off. I was accused of not being myself. I lost friendships. My family unit dissolved.

I began speaking up. I found my self-worth and reclaimed some form of self-love. I felt closer to the truth of my core than I had ever before. Every day was a challenge, but I kept choosing me.

Who decides when a woman steps into her power?

(Simple answer) She does!

For five excruciating years, I have committed to the daily devotional practice of remembering who the fuck I am.

Confronted with a new paradigm of single parenting, healing from emotional and sexual abuse, unemployment, and at one point having no real place to call my home. It was a lot!

I could have quite easily chosen to stay on that different path, one that allowed me to stay numb to experiences, or avoid my shadowy depths.

But I didn't want to miss out on the magic!

I longed for all of the juicy joy and prosperity that is offered up by the universe when we make the radical reclamation of believing in ourselves.

I choose to believe that life can be coloured with my own flavour of magic each and every day. Guided by intuition and heart, rather than obligation and judgement. I believe in manifesting dreams and leading by example for three incredible human beings that have the world at their fingertips.

There is no plan, no rules and no attachment to how things *should* look. Just the promise to use loving language towards myself, have gratitude for my body, my cycles and emotions. I accept that there will still be exhausting days, and shitty days I'd rather not endure.

Having a solid understanding of these peaks and troughs gives us a leverage point to leap back into the amazing days in full receivership.

One mentor of mine likened life to the waves of a heartbeat; *"If your life doesn't go up and down...it's flat lining, is that how you want to be existing? Is that an acceptable way for you to show up for yourself? Taking no risks? Feeling no joy?"*

Those words hit me hard and changed my whole outlook. I've learned to utilise those downward days to acknowledge all of the accomplishments that have taken place already. A humble point of reflection, an edge from which to create dreams and set goals ready to propel myself back into that next upward leap! It holds me responsible and keeps accountable for my own choices.

"You are brave..."

This is something I hear often from friends and followers watching from the sidelines, cheering me on (or not, sometimes!)

The word bravery conjures images of a Nordic Shield Maiden. Bloodied with runes drawn on her translucent skin in ritual from the sacrifice offered to the Gods, as she readies herself for battle. And a gaze that would surely pierce the hearts of her enemies.

"What is it that causes you to believe I am brave?" I have asked of those offering me this badge. Why am I like the Shield Maiden?

The reply is always variations of the same thing. I show up for myself. I take action with my goals and dreams. I don't surrender to fear, or lose faith after failure. I just keep fucking going, doing, creating.

Can I just say, for the record? Although my actions appear courageous, I don't think there has ever been a day since embarking on this *awakening* (insert other pretentious spiritual wank word here), that I haven't felt the claws of fear scratching around my throat and chest. I feel the churning in my belly, the goosebumps on my skin and I hear the negative whining of the saboteur, sitting bitterly in the back of the old English tavern with the thatched roof and low beams; pnce the life of the party and now, luring me over to their low lit corner trying to win my heart, with tales of old heartbreak and misery. The comforting voice of an old friend, who forgot how to live.

The difference? I no longer allow fear to stop me, or squash me. Sometimes I will listen to the saboteur and give them the benefit of the doubt, but I've learned that one hundred percent of the time, those old fear stories being rattled off are just a designer subconscious program that has spent the best part of 34 years trying to keep me safe.

It's just a habit that (with a little work) can be changed, altered and adapted at any time.

And once I learned that I didn't need fear programs to keep me safe *(and that … drum roll … I already am safe!)* I allowed myself to explore new horizons and take gentle risks.

I've learned to lean in to fear and perhaps even enjoy it?

In fact, you might say I have adopted somewhat of a kink relationship to fear … the more I feel it, the harder I push myself to manifest the dream or achieve the goal.

Fear is my bitch.

We are not owned by our stories. Instead, we can choose to harness the wisdom and the lessons from our experiences. As another mentor of mine says "instead of projecting blame or fear onto others for what has happened *to* us, we can make the choice to free ourselves from the attachment to those experiences and choose to honour how they have happened *for* us!"

Can you feel how this immediately changes the energy from a victim mindset into self responsibility?

"Take a lover who looks at you like maybe you are magic." – Marty McConnell

Navigating intimate relationships from an empowered space is incredibly liberating and freeing. Gone are the days when you have to give up your sense of self in order to submit to your *better half.* In fact, gone are the days you feel anything less than whole and complete *on your own!*

Being able to stand in that space and honestly feel and believe in your own magnificence is such a fucking gift.

And … side note, this embodiment makes you so incredibly sexy and desirable!

I'm not saying that my current relationship is perfect, but right now it cultivates the perfect medicine needed for our growth, both as individuals and as a couple. And for as long as it does this, I'm all in!

Having committed to a journey of self-healing and therefore remembering self-worth, my power and how to love myself, I no longer need to be saved or validated by a lover. Instead, we are able to bring more of that love to enhance our lives together, rather than manipulation, projection and clinging to feel safe.

On the flip side, I'm done trying to save men who are lost in a pile of their own shit. Oh how my heart loved someone who needed fixing, and would willingly give myself up in the process.

Nope. Not anymore.

Now I nurture, I hold and I gently poke into wounds that might need a nudge, and it is up to him whether or not he digs. He knows I am there every step of the way, but he is also aware that it's his own shit to process (if he chooses), and I'll be over here processing mine.

In truth, my heart could definitely use a little more assistance when it comes to receiving love unconditionally. I feel her disrobe and lean in to intimacy, simultaneously keeping guard to a degree. But through communication, trust and devotion to maintaining my own inner compass *(and him his)*, growth happens and love deepens.

Perception and intention is everything.

Embodying the powerful woman, does not mean that you have reached a chapter of your life wherein you are no longer faced with the potential of daily challenges.

How do you act as opposed to react to situations?

Is it a hindrance or an opportunity?

How do you choose to move through with the ease and grace of the wisdom collected like salty seashells in the pockets of a seasoned explorer?

Darling woman,

You are powerful because you got tired of being a spectator.

You are unstoppable because you kept rising.

You are worthy because there is no other flavour of magic like you in this world full of vanilla.

Embody your flavour of magic and let it drip it's sweetness onto all of those who crave a taste.

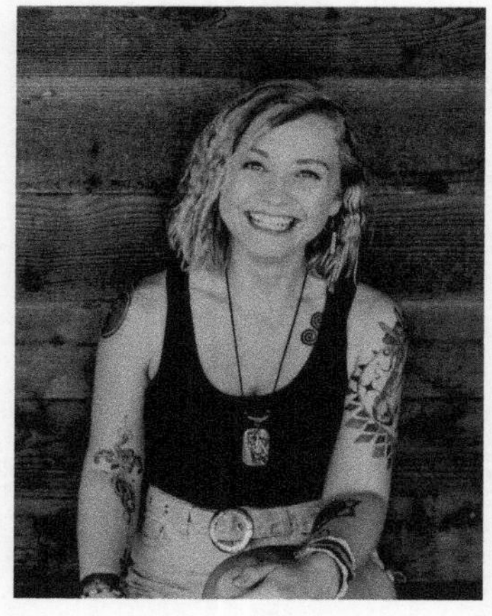

Laura Elizabeth

Hi, I'm Laura Elizabeth, a trailblazing change maker and advocate for women's empowerment. Author of Loving Herself Whole, Back Yourself! and Wild Woman Rising, creatress of Kuntea, founder of HER Centre in the rolling hills of Perth, and owner of Laura Elizabeth Wellness/Erotic Maven Medicine.

I am dedicated to creating intimate experiences for conscious women ready to step into a deeper layer of understanding of self to embrace and embody their sensuality, reclaim their voices and own their power. I offer Womb and Yoni Massage Therapy, Reiki Attunements and a catalogue of workshops, education and training online and in person.

A naturally gifted psychic medium born on the East Coast of Scotland, I moved to Perth, Western Australia, as a pre-teen in 1999. With nearly two decades of experience cultivating my skills as an energy worker and holding space for clients, I offer the safest and most profoundly intimate containers for women to encounter deep transformation.

A boundary pusher and taboo smasher, I am best known for my real, quirky and honest guidance, ensuring the deepest empathy, understanding and non-judgement.

My service to clients is most definitely a niche I believe is the real missing link in human connection and healing for women. We are programmed to think, feel, and do based on the needs of others. But we unleash our real magic when we set aside time to explore honouring, nurturing and loving ourselves back into a belief of radical acceptance and remembering our magnificence.

A passionate mother of three, leading by example, smashing goals and living with purpose, I hope to be a positive influence and for my own children to reach their full potential and inspire others to do the same.

I hold your hand and love you, while you remember how to love yourself.

www.lauraelizabeth.com.au
Instagram: @eroticmaven_medicine & @kuntea_by_le
Facebook: eroticmavenmedicine

The Art of Devotion

ASH

My knowing has always been there. My belief in myself bore a slow death as I transitioned from maiden to motherhood, wilting with each pleasure I gave away. Until I found myself so far from anything that resembled who I was, I had no choice but to begin the slow and sacred journey home.

I know exactly why it is we don't believe the whispers of our bodies; the inner callings that are here to guide us safely through our passage. I tell myself it is the journey of being human, of living this human experience. It is easier than acknowledging the truth, which is, we are suppressed, manipulated and filled with fear for living in our light. Living in our light is living in our pleasure, embracing the fullest expressions of who we are as women. Divine Goddesses, life givers, nurturers, mystics, healers, witches, medicine women, creators and guides - the Feminine is connection to Source, to The Divine. Language limits us so please take my words as my expressions. You too will find yours - certain experiences, interactions, words, people, will create a ripple within you. An expansion, a burst of lightness and energy, that the more you pay attention to the louder it will become. An empowered woman emanates Rapture, an encapsulating vibration that infiltrates the collective consciousness empowering those who are lucky enough to receive her radiance.

Yes, I believe in a collective consciousness; one that Einstein made theories on and modern science is quickly observing. The Quantum Field: I can feel the life force that flows within me, a source we all can tap into, and create a relationship with.

I am the EleMental Alchemist, I am 36 years young and gracefully embracing all of who I am as a woman, a mother, the many facets that make me, me. I find my healing in my practice, a Devotion I have discovered within me that calls me home. Back into my body, listening, honouring, being human and allowing myself to experience all of what it is to be a woman. It is here I began to really know myself, to build a relationship with myself again, and again, and again. It is here I discovered the tools that worked for me, that allowed me to relate consciously with myself so as to see a deeper depth of awareness. I learnt how to shine light on the darker aspects that had previously been kept hidden, in fear of offending others - as if it was somehow my personal responsibility to regulate others emotions.

My practice allows for the natural cyclic nature of death and rebirth, creating an awareness that allows for acceptance and action; acceptance of ones external influences, alongside ones connection to the results of powerful action. Powerful action that brings forth breakdowns that lead to breakthroughs, self-discoveries that give me greater power in choosing my way in each moment.

To me this is living a life of Empowerment. Fully choosing in each and every moment the direction we are heading. Choosing our priorities, our children, our relationships. Choosing to find our path back to our certainty and inner calm. To knowing our needs, chasing our desires and awakening our pleasures. Choosing to honour ourselves just as much as we honour those in our lives. Living a life that is our personal calling, for it is here we feel most alive, most at home. It is here we live in alignment with our values and the filling of our cup, making ourselves a priority, becomes simplified and more importantly enjoyable.

A woman alive in her pleasure oozes sensuality and grace, honouring her body for the temple it is. She is felt, seen, and heard. I have not always believed this was within me. It was awakened by other women who were reclaiming their pleasure, as we sat in sister circle. The feeling was one of coming home, of knowing with all certainty this was what I had been searching for my whole life, and perhaps many lifetime's before.

The ways of the original custodians of This Earth have slowly been bled out. Massacred with each aboriginal tribe that was slaughtered by the unhealthy expression of a patriarchal society running on greed and domination. We have forgotten our softness, we have forgotten to dance bare foot on the earth, our hips have become stiff, holding our stored emotions, we have forgotten the power held within our temple.

The past few hundred years we have slowly had our powers taken away. We are so far from ourselves, and our wisdoms, many of us now willingly hand our power to others without conscious thought.

The honour of receiving a woman in her rapture gave me an embodied understanding of Reverence. The human form with all its stories, perceptions and preconceived judgements is cleared and a woman's Divine Essence is felt and received. I have come to understand this exchange between sisters as a transmission, and these exchanges are fundamentally an awakening. It is not through language we understand, it is through feeling. A woman in her rapture raises her vibration; this is felt even when the concept is not consciously understood.

This sense of self-knowing did not come without an exchange. For every woman has her story. Most have walked a path of pleasing others, dimming their light and turning down their radiance. Most have suffered at the expense of societal limitations and perceptions. A woman's pleasure is often placed last to the pleasures of others.

The path of reclamation is a path of self-discovery. The women who speak to me do so through their rapture, the courage they show when walking their path to redemption. My sisters, who have endured things no human should ever have to endure, who are courageously stoking their internal flame whilst remembering to stoke the inner flames of their sisters (and brother's). Breaking the chains of suffering, as it is through our suffering, we awaken, we remember.

We are in a world seeking to regain its balance; a patriarchal existence that has seen the demise of the worshipping of the goddess. The feminist movement sent ripples of confusion into the relationships between men and women. Over time we have lost our connection to the earth, it's medicine and the wisdoms found within nature and within ourselves.

Those who are aware of the limitations within society, quickly find it to be a lonely road. When walking a life of fully choosing, the Rising Matriarch's who have a conscious thought, have it quickly squashed with the projections of fear from those we love, and those we trust. It takes a very powerful woman to stand her ground against her family, against the system, to stand her ground, in her knowing when all others fail to see and worship the Divine Feminine that lies before them. When those around them live not only in fear of the Divine, they are blind to it - because they have not yet remembered the Divine within themselves.

You see society fears the Divine Feminine. She is Too Loving, and we as a society do not know how to fully receive this love. She is Too Wise, and god-forbid a woman have more knowing than you. This knowing even more incomprehensible, when it defies logic. She is Too Sensual in her expression - for society does not know how to honour sensuality without wanting to claim it as their own, devouring the sacredness of sensuality, and turning it into something that resembles shame. She is far Too Courageous, for the empowered woman defies all these assumptions, she remembers, and in this remembering she continues to gain strength, she continues to find her softness. A shift of focus towards the evidence she needs to trust her body once again.

As a young girl I was naive and innocent, thinking back there were already signs of ancestral trauma in the realms of sex and sexuality. When in private places of pleasure and desire, my mind taking me to visions of being violently dominated and violated. For this reason I never explored myself in ways I needed to. It has taken me twenty-five years to acknowledge this part of myself. Knowing what I know now, I had very little hope of growing into my power and embodying all of who I was in a linear trajectory. After all, an Empowered Woman is a woman connected to her pleasure. An empowered woman is a woman who embraces all of who she is, sensual, sexual, wild, knowing and untamable, until she herself chooses to tame her wild and thus bring balance and harmony into existence.

This is where the problem lies, as society is looking to tame us all. This is where we lost our power.

I assume our story is similar to many of yours, with slightly different details. The theme the same. What I also assume is that every family has its own story. Children are raised in families where parents fail to acknowledge and validate their own emotions. This has a ripple effect and we fail to acknowledge and validate the emotions of our children. A need to fix, turn down and turn off ones emotions has a profound effect resulting in patterns and behaviours that serve to protect as a young child - and become dysfunctional as we grow into adolescents and adults.

The Rise of the Matriarch is one of discovering the strength in our softness. Remembering the Power in Vulnerability, Receptivity and acts of Devotion; truth and the telling of our stories from a place where we have moved through our rage and come back to love.

My own mother crushed my spirit many times over. Perhaps the most poignant, was the time I first gained the courage to speak about my relationship. It had taken five years for me to unblock the memories; five years for me to build the courage within me to speak my experiences out loud.

I found myself in her kitchen, skimming the surface as to the depth of my pain and the reasons for my tears; I was feeling shamed in my parenting for the behaviours of my children. I wasn't good enough. My children weren't good enough. I was finding reasons for their behaviour. I had started to put the dots together, recognising the dysfunctional behaviours - as the dysfunctional behaviours that were also within me. Sharing snippets of my own experiences and drawing parallel lines to the behaviours of my children.

Confusion.

An inability to make a decision.

Self Doubt.

Self Loathing.

Stomach Problems from Stress.

You see we bore the same role. Serve and Nurture. Do not be seen, or heard, and definitely do not have your own opinion or desires.

The path of the Wounded Healer I have come to understand.

My mothers programmed reaction revealed to me just how dysfunctional our society (and my family) was. My own mother, who bore witness to my pain, my sadness, had not seen her own grandchildren and daughter as much as should have been.

My mother's words did not crush me that day, for my soul had exited my body many years before, and many times over. My mother's words were short and simple, a moment in time I will never forget, for with these words the Matriarch within me stood a little higher, her whispers came a little louder.

Her words awakened an even deeper certainty within me. An even stronger pull towards knowing this was NOT ok. This journey I was travelling was not one any of the recent women in my family had travelled before me. I was on this journey alone; there would be no elders to hold me in my suffering, no elders to guide me back to wholeness, there would be no guidance, safety or holding from those I sought these safeties in. For none before me had reclaimed their fullness, none had walked the path back home to themselves, to the vast array of pleasures, emotions and magic that lie within them. They may have tasted droplets of their power, when birthing their babes, as small flutters of remembering, felt as unexplainable knowing's that came from deep in their bones. They however, failed to follow their callings.

It was then that I knew - no matter how many times I shared, no matter how many stories I told, I would still be seen as the one telling stories. I would still be seen as the one playing victim.

So once again I stopped sharing my story. Once again I held my pain inside. Once again I smiled outwardly and died inwardly. Once again the disconnection grew, the misunderstanding grew, and the support lessened. No wonder we turn away from receiving help.

Somehow, somewhere, I found deep within me, a strength to love harder and heal my wounds; to feel the pains that flowed within my blood, passed down to my children. I fought not for me, but for them and their right to live abundantly, full of lust and vitality. My journey through motherhood driving me further into my own pain.

As my journey took course, it became clear this was not just my journey, but one of all sisters and brothers, through all lineages - the men and woman of our lands, our blood and the blood of our ancestors who walked these lands before us. The time is Now.

I found the strength to travel to the depths of my darkness. The places I kept hidden. The places I had learnt to shame, hide and forget. To feel the pain in my body from not only my lifetime, but from my mothers, and her mothers -

and her mothers. The suffering and silencing that began as the Matriarch was burned and the Patriarch was built. We are the generation that is here to create change. WE are the generation that is acknowledging the imbalances, the hurts and the failures, without placing blame externally.

We are holding our own, and by fuck it is a lonely journey.

An empowered woman is desired by many, and feared by even more, for an empowered woman reflects back to you the parts of yourself you are trying not to see.

In 2017 I chose powerfully with my intentions. I had attended a taster evening for a woman's circle called Dancing Eros. I knew this was where I needed to be, this was the circle of women I had been seeking my whole life, and probably many lifetimes before.

It began that evening as I sat in circle with sisters, as I heard their moans and groans in pleasure and in grief. It began as I embodied my Wild and allowed the energies of the Witches to curse through my being, awakening my ability to take what I need. It began as I slowed down my breath, simplified my touch, and realised just how numb my physical body was to receiving any sort of pleasure led by me, for me. After a very uncomfortable evening of self seduction and self discovery, asked if I would be attending the Immersion - I answered immediately and without thought

"Ill find a way."

The power of our Pussy and a woman who is listening to the whispers of her body and it's needs.

Ok.

I was ready. I knew where I needed to be, and I knew I needed to reclaim my Pussy and all of its juicy pleasures. I was angry at all that had been taken away. I was angry at the men in my family. I was angry at my exes. I was angry at the world in which we live and make these things acceptable, normal.

NYE saw me practicing simple ritual and magic and manifesting the return of my pleasure. I knew there was more to receive, and I knew I was being triggered in my intimate relationship. I had awakened the beast - and she was not calming down until I listened.

The leader of the Immersion released a competition, the universe was listening and answered my prayers, I won. I would be attending the five-day Immersion as a gift. The following is one of my first reflections:

Driving to day 3 of our Dancing Eros Immersion.

Reflecting on my most vulnerable state.

Vulnerable?

I do not allow myself to be vulnerable.

I am strong.

I am capable.

I cannot afford to be vulnerable.

Vulnerability is weakness… or so I had come to believe.

I was witnessing the subtle power in others softness. I was awakening to the concept that my desires were on the other side of my vulnerabilities. Perhaps I needed to lean into these edges, perhaps I needed to find a way to be received in my grief. My memories of those years were vast and non-existent.

I began to block out my pain in childhood, with a strong and independent mother, an imbalance of the logical, goal driven, independent Yang energy …

This was quite beneficial for the most part as a young strong youth.

As I began my transition to motherhood at the young age of 19, as my pregnancy grew, the wounds of our childhood were thrown into the spotlight. A deep-rooted sadness began to form within my body.

The loneliness

The confusion

The questions

The silent tears alone in the darkness. The numbing. The blocking of my pain - which I now understand was the blocking of my pleasure, and thus my power.

As I find a way to acknowledge the little girl within me, and all of her feelings, as I bring back the pain and sadness, I begin to find a way to feel safe within my body. I create the container and learn how to move these emotions and energies through me. No longer attached to the emotions I feel arise within me.

I am so blessed to have heard the whispers and followed their callings. To have started my journey towards my true authentic self, the fullest expression of me, all parts of me. The soft and the hard. The receptive and the assertive. The Creatrix and the Destroyer. The calm and the chaos. To all the women who are claiming all aspects of themselves, I see you. Continue upon this journey you find yourself on. Take this as no coincidence you find yourself reading these words. Follow that inner calling that guides you. Honour your truest essence.

As the tears flow and I let them roll to the edge of my cheek, the thoughts start. The memories. Recognition to my journey and all I have experienced.

Over the years I have come to know my most vulnerable state is in admitting my story, and coming to believe that this does not make me unworthy.

My body is my body.

My pleasure is my pleasure, and this is my birthright.

To express the depth of my grief and sadness is not to place blame, or to call victim.

It is simply to feel, so as we can begin to heal. Finding our way back to Devotion, where we can see Divinity within us all.

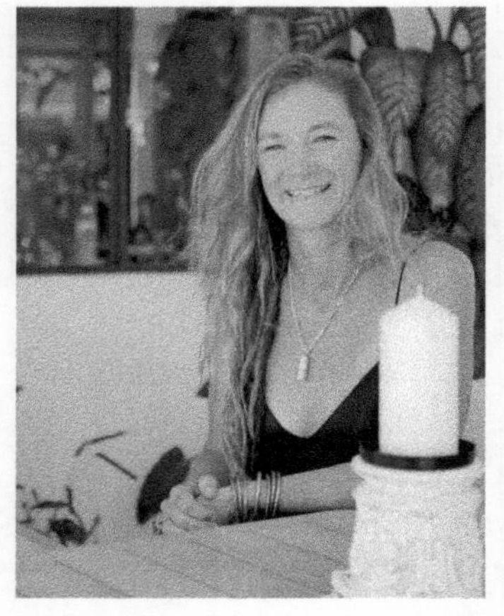

ASH

My name is Aimee Sullivan Hamilton, and I am no longer afraid of the vast array of emotions that flow through me. I welcome all parts of me, and I use my body as the powerful vessel it is to express, transmute and create.

My desires guide me, welcoming me to places previously feared and uncertain. Now, the certainty I seek comes from within, a current that flows within and with out.

Life is my practice, living has become my rituals. I find myself listening to the medicine of the birds as their song catches my attention, receiving wisdoms from their flight, creating more and more space in the everyday, to receive the answers I seek.

I hold space for grief, death and the decaying. For it is on the other side of these challenges one finds praise, rebirth & devotion. I hold space.

I hold space for that which is messy, wild & often euphoric.

I am becoming known as the EleMental Alchemist, for I work closely with the natural world, plants, animals, nature spirits and of course - the elements. Together we remind others how to come home to their bodies. Home to the wisdoms held in the spaces between the noise. Together we invite the remembering, allowing others to find their safe container to feel.

As we learn to feel, we can begin to heal - and from this place we can begin to understand ourselves from a different perspective. We can journey deep into the unknown because we have the container to FEEL SAFE.

Certainty is a human need that is essential in times such as these.

2020 saw a year like no other in modern times.

Are you being called home? To your greatest certainty, found within the subtle sensations that awaken within your body the more you turn inwards.

The more you listen, and begin to discern the whisperings.

Welcome home, sweet child.

ASH

www.aimee-hamilton.com
Email: movement4life@outlook.com
Instagram: @movement4life_
Bch Sports & Exercise Science
Master Practitioner Hypnosis
Master Life Coach (mum-preneurs)
Wildgrace Initiatress
Yoga Teacher

Limitless, Fearless, Fierce

Amanda Greasley

For me, the matriarch conjures images of the grumpy old governess, stalking the halls of a boarding school, making sure no one is breaking the rules and imposing her stern and cross energy over anyone who dares step near her. For others, the matriarchy symbolises the ugly side of the women's liberation movement; triggering fears of women taking power away from men and throwing them into the depths of subservience.

The Rising of the Matriarch represents the Rising of the Mother for me. The mother archetype needs no love in return, for she receives her love through the giving of love. By pouring her love into every crevice of all things, she nurtures all creation, including herself, and shifts the world from fear into love. But along with the love is a fierceness that cannot be ignored. Like our Mother Gaia, the mother archetype is wild, untamed, breathtakingly beautiful, raw, fierce, soft and nourishing. She embodies the balance of all things and gifts us with each side of the scale in every moment, love in the absence of fear, death in the absence of life.

She knows what you need; whether it is a love filled embrace that melts into every cell of your body, or a harsh serve of tough love that smacks you into last year - she always seems to know.

My own mother embodies this mother archetype and she raised strong, independent and courageous daughters. She has been my inspiration for as long as I can remember and fills me with so much pride I feel my heart may break open and flood the world with soul-soothing, spirit-lifting, life-affirming energy. Knowing her, watching her and learning from her is what gave me the courage to both embrace and embody the mother within me, and there have been so many times in my grown life where I have leaned into that energy to facilitate significant change.

I grew up with complicated beliefs about myself. I was so self-conscious; worried about what other people thought of me and terrified of displeasing anyone, regardless of the cost to myself. I felt picked on and singled out, or ignored and looked over. I wanted only to be one of the cool kids and to be accepted by my peers, but had very little belief in myself; that's how I remember it as a grown-up anyway. I was the uncool kid hanging out with the cool kids; never really belonging. I was too fat, too boring, not pretty enough, I didn't have cool clothes and was often told that if I wanted to do well in life I needed to focus and apply myself, and stop day-dreaming.

I don't think it was a life too different from many other kids growing up, but I did at the time, and my suitcase of negative self-beliefs travelled with me, until I was well into my late thirties.

It was in my late twenties, that I realised I owned this suitcase. I had just lost my job and the car that came with the position, had no savings, no relationship and my friendships were only just holding on.

Four years prior I ended a relationship and a friendship all at once and it threw me into deep depression. I hid myself away from the world, only leaving the house for work and to occasionally see my coven sisters who loved me regardless of me living my half-life. I hated myself and judged myself fiercely. I stacked on weight and had numerous unrequited loves, who probably had no idea I even thought of them in that way. I had no confidence and a whole gamut of unhelpful beliefs about myself and the world. If I ever dared to dream about a different life, I would hate on myself.

No one will love you, you're too fat

No one will love you, you're too boring

No one will love you, you've been alone too long

You have nothing worthwhile to offer anyone

I really didn't see myself very clearly at all and I lived that way for a little over eight years.

It wasn't all bad during those years of solitude. I got a new job in a new industry under a brilliant, fierce and business-minded powerhouse of a woman; she taught me so much about friendship, leadership and being a woman in power in a male-dominated industry. I think the most important thing she did for me in the four years I worked for her, was to acknowledge my intellect and my commitment. She gave me courage to want more, to push the boundaries of my comfort zone – in many ways she was the catalyst for the rebirthing of my soul.

Armed with this new found and self-defined confidence, I was no longer happy to live in the shadows, and I made the decision to challenge more of my beliefs about myself and the world. Looking back, perhaps it wasn't the healthiest way to challenge myself, but I needed to do something; at twenty-eight living my life alone without adventure or love, was no longer an appealing life choice. As I reflect on it I would not change my decision for anything, but having a deeper understanding of how fear plays out in our behaviours, I can see now that I was still seeking external validation for my existence.

Insert the next adventure … online dating. Now, we're talking about online dating in 2008 where choices were limited as to how it happened (smart phones weren't a thing yet). My goal was to challenge the belief that no one would ever find me attractive, and that I didn't have anything to offer. I wanted to find myself.

There has been no other time in my life where I could so relate to a baby seal in a shark tank.

Many of the men were much older and were nothing but degrading and, to put it frankly, fucking pigs. But, as time went on, I got more 'savvy.' I learned how to play the online dating game; until I was playing it better than they were. I spent a little over a year getting to know myself, and I got my self-confidence back, albeit based on external validation. And I wouldn't change a thing. I am unashamed and a much stronger person for those months of self-exploration. I connected with my sacred feminine, I explored how she felt, how her soft energy flowed; strong enough to carve a path through stone. I fed my connection to myself. I stood strong in my power to say no and learned how to ask for what I wanted.

During this time, I also learned there is no shame in women enjoying sex or wanting to connect with another person in this way. I abhor slut shaming and the judgement that comes when a woman openly admits to being sexually liberated. I have faced that judgement many times. I have had relationships ended and strained because of it. I know who I am and I am a much stronger, braver and self-assured woman because of it. If I had shied away from this year of challenging my boundaries, in one of the most socially unacceptable ways, I would still be a hermit, hating myself and the world. I would not understand my own physical body, nor my own mind.

Sometimes the mother archetype is radical and solves problems or catalyses change in the most unexpected of ways. Like a cyclone I needed an extreme event, to take extreme action to claim back my power and my life.

Four years later I became a mother. It still amazes me how much a woman's needs change once she becomes a mother, and I really wish that this fundamental change in our makeup was explained to us at some point in time. So … if you haven't yet had a baby, please know that your needs as a woman and a mother will change. I was living my life in a relationship when really, I needed a partnership.

Even though I was a shell of a person for most of the eight years I was single, I did gain a strength of self that was perhaps the undoing of my relationship with my son's father. I remained fiercely independent; a self-preservation response to living with someone with severe anxiety and depression, and I was terrified that I was being pulled into that depression with him. Every day I would live with the uncertainty of what mood he would be in when I got home from work. Would I have to make excuses for him? There were days I left work early, because the only communication from him was "I don't know if I can go on."

When I say this may have been the undoing of the relationship, it definitely wasn't the only contributing factor. I struggled, every day, with the burden of being the only income for our family, of having to come home from work and still clean the kitchen and cook dinner. I wasn't good at asking for help, and he wasn't good at hearing me when I did. I broke down crying one night, again asking for help, but none came. I felt so burdened, so tired and weighed down, that when my son was two, I ended the relationship.

I had realised that this was not the relationship model that I wanted my son to grow up with and think was 'normal.' I realised there was no "in love" left in our relationship. Both of us were only half living and, for my son, I knew that was unacceptable. It was hard. It was so so hard, but it was the only way. Every part of the mother in me was screaming to make change, to provide the best opportunity for my son, to see how healthy relationships work, to show him partnership. It was hard and I hurt the man that I had once been in love with, but I couldn't ignore that I was hurt too, and I had been betrayed and let down by the man who was meant to love me. Sometimes I think about it and it seems so petty. I ended a relationship because he wouldn't cook or clean the kitchen, but then I remember it was because he didn't choose me. My needs were not a consideration. They weren't something that he could meet.

This was the true birthing of my mother archetype; the fierce, protective, enough is enough, no nonsense energy that I needed in the moment. I knew it was going to be difficult, but I wasn't actually prepared for the emotions and drama that ensued after the breakup. The aftermath felt harder than the action itself, but sitting in that mother energy I was able to withstand the fallout. I feel it is so important to note here now, that a few years later we get along just fine.

Life is nothing but choices. Although the consequences of that choice may not be what we want, there is always choice; even if it is how we allow an event to impact our future, our reactions or our beliefs about ourselves.

And I grieve.I cry, I numb out and I scream with Kali rage at the weight of these decisions. That when faced with disempowerment, I must make the decision to fight, to rise. I must consciously choose myself at all times. Sink or swim. I grieve that the world has so lost its connection with the divine feminine that we are rarely allowed the space to surrender to the ebb and flow of the natural cycles of life. When I reflect on these big journeys of claiming back my power, I know myself as the Warrior, the Matriarch and the Mother - strong, fierce and capable of anything. When we need to embody these archetypes, the events are life changing.

The rising of the mother, the matriarch, is the rising of empowered women. It is not the voices of crazy, women's liberation, or even women demanding equality. It is us claiming back our internal power; a strength that has been lost through generations of social and tribal expectations. It is the shedding of the "good girl" identity and the embracing of our individuality. We ebb and flow, we move in cycles, just as the seasons and our beautiful mother Gaia. We are emotional. We are messy and loud. We are unstructured and impulsive.

We are not a threat to the divine masculine, but we are a threat to the toxic masculine, for as we rise, this must fall. As the mother rises within us we will no longer accept bad treatment, silencing or abuse. We will seek partners who are unafraid of us. Partners who will support us in our rising, knowing that they too will grow along side us; partners who know we will challenge their beliefs about love, partnership and themselves.

I am still fiercely independent three years on and am in a partnership with a man who chooses me every damn day, and I choose him. I do not fear that he will take my independence; it is one of the things he most loves about me. Because I know who I am, I do not fear that he will hurt me so much I pick up that suitcase of crap and drop down into the pits of self-depreciation again. I am confident in myself and no one has the power to take that away from me. Loving myself means I can love others more fully. I can accept love and I can also accept it when love isn't on offer in that moment. Love is such a complicated emotion. Loving yourself is the only way you can fully love another.

This leads me to where I am now. I have learned how to recognise the fear within me, the bullshit negative self-beliefs, and the blocks holding me back and keeping me small. I'm reminded of something I read by author, Byron Katie. Is it love, approval or acceptance we seek from others? Knowing the answer to this question will have a significant impact on the choices we make in our lives.

Whatever your answer is is what you actually need to seek in yourself. It impacts your relationships and the decisions you make. Mine is approval; I have spent most my life seeking the approval of others. Staying small and basing my life decisions (mostly) on the fear that people won't approve of me or my choices. When I do make a decision that I feel others won't approve of, I am secretive about it and don't share it with anyone who I believe may judge me for it. I am blessed enough that I have people in my life who won't judge me regardless of what I do, but that fear does hold me back, still. And this... my chapter in this incredible book, is a huge step for me in not seeking external approval, owning my choices and decisions and standing by them. After all, it is my life, my journey and my lessons.

So now, after my huge journey in knowing who the fuck I actually am, I can honestly say that I lead the rising of empowered and soulfully connected women. Women who are catalysts for change; who want to change their lives and the lives of others in a powerful and meaningful way.

I support female disruptors in changing their *own* world, so they can then change *the* world;

the mothers, the witches, the warriors, the leaders, the women with a story, the women with a message, the women with love to give, and the women who fight for those who cannot yet fight for themselves, those who live in congruence and without fear, in love and trust, with clarity, focus and a fierce passion.

I am a catalyst for change in this world and so are you.

One of my teachers, Elisha Halpin, said in a recent training session... we want to change the world, we want the world to be a nicer place BUT we aren't making those changes in our own lives. How can we expect the world to change if we aren't willing to be the demonstration of what we want the world to be?

If I am to be a sacred leader and lead this rising of empowered change-makers then I better ensure I am being the demonstration of how I want the world to be.

So I am starting with me. I love my women empowered. I love women who know who they are and if anyone doesn't like it then, actually, that's too bad. And I don't discount the men either. I love men empowered; empowered to feel and express their emotions without fear of being shamed or not being 'manly' enough. Just as I want women to be soft but strong, I want men to be strong but soft. I want everyone to be able to express emotion in a healthy way, freely. I want everyone in this world to feel safe, regardless of their gender (birth or chosen), their race, their religion, and their socio-economic standing. I want everyone to be able to see their fears for what they are; nothing more than an absence of love. I want equality in opportunity.

I will lead this rising of empowered and soulfully connected women, who can embody the mother archetype within them and sit in the blazing fires of Kali-Ma's rage; allowing the fires to consume her and push her into revolution against injustice and inequality.

I will lead the rising of empowered and soulfully connected women who are the catalysts for change in this world. Being a catalyst for change, means being the demonstration of what you want the world to look like every day,inspiring others to be brave, to take a chance, to take a breath, to stop, just for a moment. Inspiring others to look within themselves, to know themselves and understand they are unlimited potential.

I will lead this rising of empowered and soulfully connected women, who can embody the mother archetype and pour their nectar into the wounds of this reality.

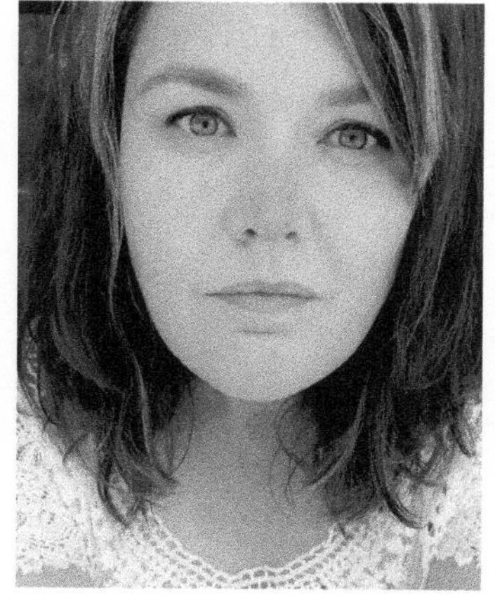

Amanda Greasley

Hi, I'm Amanda Greasley, a catalyst for change in universal consciousness, a fear huntress and founder of HER Source Pty Ltd.

I am dedicated to leading the rising of soulfully connected and empowered women; the change makers in this world. I support the female disruptors in changing their own world so they can then change the world. To live in congruence and without fear, in love and trust and with clarity, focus and a fierce passion. The Mothers, the witches, the warriors, the leaders, the women with a story, the women with a message, the women with love to give and the women who fight for those who cannot yet fight for themselves.

A qualified Intuitive Intelligence Trainer and Spiritual Leader, I was born in Perth in Western Australia. I have over 20 years experience in honing my skill as an energy worker, an intuitive and holder of sacred energy, I hold my clients safely in sacred space as they shift their limiting beliefs and fears and transmute them into love.

Quick witted and with no polka face, I am known for cutting through masks and illusion to illuminate the truth. I am non-judgemental and deeply compassionate.

My service to the World, the universal consciousness is to know myself, and guide my Clients to know themselves as limitless, fearless, fierce. To eliminate the belief of separation in the world and to encourage the belief of oneness. To know yourself as limitless, fearless, fierce means to know yourself as God (universal consciousness), to surrender to the guidance of your intuition, to honour yourself and to work in the underworld of your conscious, transmuting limiting beliefs and fear patterns into love. It is my Service to be the demonstration of what I want the world to be.

A devoted mother to four incredible children, I am the demonstration of an empowered woman for them all. An inspiration to my 2 girls and a guide to my 2 boys; I trust that my embodiment of the Mother, the Warrior, the Alchemist and the Priestess will show them the way to their fullest potential in life, love and spirituality.

I am unafraid for you and hold you with the deepest compassion as you journey to knowing yourself as limitless, fearless, fierce.

www.hersource.com.au
Instagram: @her_source-intuition
Facebook: amandagreasleyhersource

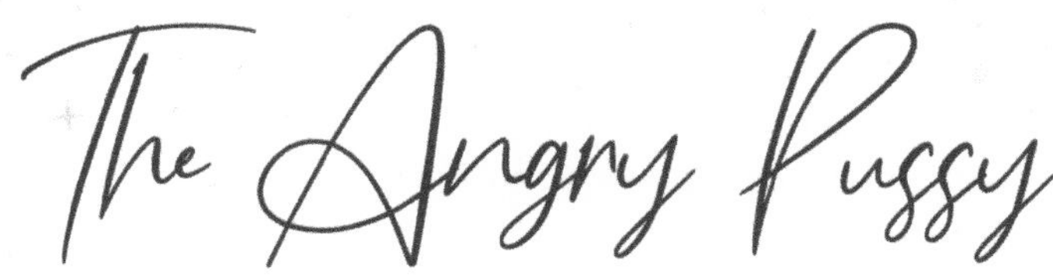

Ashamed & Unexpressed

Amberlee Carney

A Journey Through Rage to Find Purpose, Pleasure and Power.

A woman in her power, her true wild feminine power, is only deeply terrifying to the great and powerful Oz.

Those who gained and held power through the illusion of smoke and mirrors. Whose power was taken by force and control, through bribery and corruption. Creating an elaborate ruse, fooling us into believing our power lay outside of ourselves, needing to be earnt.

His fear was so strong that we began to fear our own power.

He burned our witch ancestors, casting his own dark spell putting us deep into a slumber of forgetting. Consumed by the fear that we might wake up. We might just remember and he will lose it all. Trembling at the thought that we might reveal the hurt, lost, little boy masquerading as supreme authority and power. Dreading the day we shine a light on the darkest parts of self he has been running away from for so long.

What happens if we find out there is nothing to earn?

That there is no power that could live outside of us?

That the power of all creation lies within us?

Each obstacle and challenge was beginning to feel like an initiation, opening me to one undeniable truth. That all this time, my power laid right there, between my thighs.

All this time I had been told I was inferior, been judged and shamed for being a woman. I was made to feel weak and in search of perfection to earn respect and worthiness. Made to fear my period, pleasure, birth, menopause - anything to do with my pussy.

I found my power in my connection with my womb, my feminine emotional body and my sexuality and pleasure.

There is no way I could have predicted that my path to healing my own depression and embodying self-love was through getting hands deep into pussy.

If you have arrived at this chapter, and have continued to read past my introduction I trust that you are or will be journeying with the dark goddess soon, the wild woman or connecting to the Great Mother. I trust that your soul has been yearning to open to deeper and more intimate ways of expressing yourself and your essence. That the rising of the goddess has awakened an awareness to your relationship with your body, with your sexuality, with all of the hidden and suppressed parts of self. Like me, you've heard her call and you are being initiated into a deeper truth. One that no longer separates us from the forces of nature, one that is heart and womb centred, one that honours that we all came from the divine mother and we will all return to her.

***

This work, this chapter included, has been bringing to light every single part of me that isn't in full integrity yet.

The places where I have been pretending to be powerless and where I was giving my power away.

The moments in which I hid behind blame, weak excuses, or ran away.

It has been ugly, uncomfortable, painful but so fucking necessary.

Holding space for myself to feel the gravity of every part of my being that has been acting out of integrity with my truth without falling into the fit of shame, judgement, self-pity and self-hatred has been an incredible indicator of my growth.

I had been listening to myself speak about embracing and loving all parts of my emotional and wild self, but then judging and chastising myself in private.

Demanding trust, love and abundance from the universe, but then still filtering myself through a lens of fear.

I was yearning for the fullness of the feminine. I wanted all of her delectable gifts. I wanted my soul's purpose and passion. Something deep within my womb stirred and longed for liberation.

I wasn't prepared for the intensity in which I would feel again. The embodied feminine path strips you bare and forces you to feel *everything*.

That sensitivity I was shamed for as a child? It just grew tenfold. All of the layers that kept me separate, armoured and numb were getting ferociously peeled back and, without any protection, I was anxious about the magnitude in which I would be able to feel before physically breaking apart.

There is no hiding from yourself here. She forces you to visit the deepest, most hidden parts of self. That is what the dark is, not the bad, not the evil, just the hidden, the deep and the mysterious. All so you can see where you need to direct more love. So you can integrate each part and love yourself back into wholeness.

***

Initially, I struggled with the term matriarchy. It left a bad taste in my mouth.

Power to me had been distorted, competitive, controlling, forceful, oppressive.

A struggle that was causing resistance to this chapter. Resistance to matriarchal truth and power. I kept picking at the scab. What was there? I was looking for a golden thread in my journals, meditation, breathwork, self-pleasure, anywhere! *I've had it! I'm done! I have no story!*

It wasn't that I had *no* story. It was that I didn't want to tell *this* story. The pages of my journal were screaming at me with unrelenting anger towards my motherline, my mother and my grandmother. Rage engulfed me. But it didn't make sense and I felt nauseating shame and guilt over it.

Yes, I had been working on accepting all parts of myself, every emotion, but I had unleashed something that felt uncontrollable and ill-directed.

I was angry at my motherline for being so fucking small.

Filled with indignation for them being keepers of such intuitive gifts and spiritual knowledge yet never healing themselves. Judgemental, opinionated, always advising, never listening. Never apologising, never admitting when they're wrong. Buying into the patriarchal bullshit and using control and power over, instead of finding their own power and strength within. Hiding and suppressing emotions, becoming guarded and unapproachable.

Resentful that they were too scared, too fearful to do this inner work themselves. Not leading the way. Not showing me how to connect to myself, my bleed, my power as a woman. Never showing me how to love myself or that I am worthy of love. Thoughtlessly instilling more fear into me about being a vulva owner in her power.

This rage served me in a way as all rage does. It showed me where I don't want to be. Who I don't want to be. It showed me where I had had enough. What I no longer wanted to carry in my matriarchal line.

But it also protected something deeper than that. It became a shield, a veil covering my own need for rightness, blaming them for all this painful work that I *had* to do because they chose not to. The choice I felt was taken away because *they* didn't make that choice before me. Because *they* followed in the footsteps of fear.

Anger became protection for where I was putting myself into powerlessness.

My ego was using this anger to hide from the responsibility of stepping into my power.

Responsibility for the consequences of being in my power. What would I have to change? What would I have to let go of? The fear of having to step into this power alone. Angry they weren't holding me, supporting me and journeying with me.

Spiritually immature and deep in my victimhood. I didn't want to see that in myself.

I was protecting myself from seeing how fucking arrogant and entitled I was being.

Angry that I have to break this for my line? I don't *have* to do anything at all. I *get* to stand up and break this for future generations. Women before me have suffered immensely so that I *get* to heal the feminine wounding. I *get* to break patriarchal chains. I *get* to choose a life of personal and sexual liberation. And I *get* to ignite this fire in the world for all women.

This hit hard. It was explosive. Bursting through my chest. Love, compassion and forgiveness flooded my heart. It was fierce and full-bodied. A breakthrough that allowed me to finally acknowledge and celebrate my mother's strength and resilience. Leaving her first husband to protect my older sister. Just a baby at the time. The breaking point was when he hit her in the face, breaking her tooth with my sister in her arms. My grandmother described the blood still on the ceiling from the incident. This is when she said enough.

Then I felt it. Waves of unexpressed, suppressed rage washing over my body. No one to witness or hold space for this magnitude of emotion. There was a certainty in every cell of my being. The rage I had been feeling was hers.

I wailed. A guttural moan I have only heard from myself a few times in my life which accompanied unbearable grief. I felt with complete truth in my body that this rage was for her. She is more courageous than I will ever know. She fought these demons so that I will never have to. She made a choice that was completely in her power. I dropped into the feelings of shame around being in an abusive relationship. Feeling disempowered and dishonoured. I felt a lifetime of judgement, of feeling unloved and unseen, reflected in her.

A second surge of anger as I felt the betrayal from a man who was supposed to be good, kind and safe. This time staying in this disempowered position for her three children. Safe and secure. This anger was wild, unexpressed, uncontrollable. It had been buried. With guilt and shame, it had been buried. When you bury a rage like this it either turns inwards, into bitterness and resentment, or it explodes and isn't conscientious about what is destroyed in its path.

I had welcomed the fire, but I didn't expect it to be the medicine in healing my relationship with my mother. I am not angry at her. I am angry with her. This is her rage. This is the rage of the collective feminine. I will not dim the fire of my anger. Honouring this anger will free me from generational pain and suffering. It will burn the shackles of the patriarchy, of conditioned beliefs in separation, of the demonisation of our sexuality and intuition.

***

As women, we have been shamed for anger, for wrath. We've been told she is a sin.

We must hold it in, we must accept what is happening to us.

Take it lying down. Passive and submissive.

A "good girl" may feel anger but she certainly must not show it.

Looking at it now, it makes sense my path to healing my motherline wounds was through healing what was considered most taboo. Accepting and loving rage. Exploring the profound mysteries of the dark feminine. Healing through sacred sexuality. Lilith, wild woman, demoness, seductress, dark goddess, made a perfect guide into loving these intense and unaccepted emotions. Honouring them with curiosity and love.

It was always going to be Earthy. Dark. Tumultuous.

Embodying Lilith ignited my own rage for the patriarchy and feminine wounding. Scorned and shunned.

Holding onto this deep-rooted archetypal fear that if I displease you, I will be exiled and replaced with an easier, more subservient, pleasing version of woman.

If I demand to be seen as an equal. If I own my desires and pleasure.

If I ask you to lay beneath me so I may revel in my own ecstasy and yours.

If I claim my birthright I will be raped. I will be thrown out. I will be threatened. My children will be murdered. I will be misconstrued as a demoness who seduces helpless men and kills babies.

No, owning my power and claiming my equality on this earth has never been safe.

I didn't need anyone to tell me this directly. I learnt it through the world, and it is reinforced every day through a world that says I am inferior on this earth for owning a vulva. The face of Lilith.

I feel her with me. Ferocious. Wild. Erotic.

"I was made of this earth and you somehow think this makes me inferior to you? Like I am here just to serve you? To please you? For you to use me and dispose of me?

No. No, I will not have it. No more. Enough."

As I practised loving and accepting myself in this state I cultivated enough safety in my feeling body to keep picking at this wound. This fear of being seen as a powerful and sexual woman was irrational. I was not going to be severely punished, ostracised, raped or killed in this lifetime for owning my voice, my unique expression and taking up space ~~in this lifetime~~. This fear, this pain was in my blood, in my DNA, it lingered in my womb. Generations of women before me had stayed safe by keeping quiet, complacent, small, by suppressing their feminine magic and mystery. They hushed and denied their daughters magic to keep them safe too.

Reminding myself that I *get* to do this work, I let Lilith's fire burn and transmute these fears into healing and liberation for all. They weren't mine. But I was still scared to be seen as an Erotic Maven, a Priestess, a Pussy Witch. What *was* real for me in this lifetime then?

The fear of being ridiculed, judged and shamed for the work I am doing. Holding temple space for sexual healing and awakening. A proud advocate for womb wisdom, periods, pleasure and pussy power. I feared being deeply misunderstood and rejected. That I would always be an outsider and no one would truly understand me. This sounded like a lonely place. With this core wounding and fear do you not think I would have chosen an easier path to awakening if there was one for me? A less risky and less taboo career? A life where I was guaranteed I would be accepted and loved by all?

I couldn't ignore the remembering of truth and power I felt in every single cell of my body when I heard the goddess call. I was afraid of this unexplained knowing that I had done this work before, that it was Truth, but I couldn't ignore it. I have learnt to trust that my body is my greatest teacher and healer. Yoni connection would be my medicine.

***

I pulled back the white cotton sheets to see a small patch of dark red blood. It was the final yoni massage I was to receive during this training in Bali. Safe in the hands of a Medicine Womban I trusted to hold, honour and love me during my bleed, the very woman who has held and nurtured this book. I surrendered into her grace and journeyed as she unlocked deep codes of feminine wisdom buried deep within my body with her intention and magical hands.

This was the first time I met her. The Great Mother, Gaia. Papatuanuku.

She was fierce and beautiful. She was fire and water. She was wild, untamed, unapologetic and yet there was nothing I would change about her. A majestic force of nature.

I had no desire to control her, cage her, tell her how to create, how to move.

I saw her as nothing other than sacred. So inextricably connected to us.

Then I felt her sorrow, her inextricable pain and devastation. Her volcanic, unfathomable rage. How we had been abusing her, exploiting her, polluting her without any sense of remorse or grief. Treating her as if she was not a living breathing entity and soul that was providing us with sustenance to live and thrive. We had been treating her as if she were inferior to us.

Using her. Dismissing her. With no respect for her, no sense of our deep interconnected relationship with her, we separated ourselves from her.

I felt a deep reconnection of my feminine soul to my body.

A homecoming.

Do you feel the connection here sister? The reflection in the mirror? This is how the patriarchy has been treating the feminine soul. They are not separate. Reclaiming my truth and power? This meant remembering that I am connected, pussy to earth. I am divine. I am sacred. I am a priestess. A witch. A wild woman. It is my birthright to be honoured, loved and revered.

I will not be shamed, domesticated and no longer will I anaesthetise myself in fear of my own power.

This was just the briefest of meetings into my multifaceted feminine soul reflected in the Great Mother. Unfurling, unravelling, unleashing the innate truth stored in my body of who I truly am. Without obligations, without pleasing others. Reintegrating all of the rejected parts of self that had been buried for lifetimes.

This was only one yoni massage. But it unlocked a power I cannot deny any longer. It shifted me forever. It confirmed my purpose in the world that would pain me to ever shy away from again.

I am here to use my voice, to make noise, to shake others from their fear-based patterns.

I am here to welcome in, love and celebrate the hidden parts of the feminine that have been demonised, suppressed and shamed for distorted power.

I, Amberlee Rose Carney, am here to initiate women into their true nature, as cyclical, powerful, mystical, sexual beings.

You, gorgeous woman, are sacred. You deserve all the bliss, ecstasy and pleasure life has to offer. This is your birthright.

Do you know what is most terrifying about a woman in her full power?

It's not really because she can't be fucked with. It's not even because she embraces all that is natural, wild, messy and erotic. What is most terrifying about being around a woman in her true power is that she will make you uncomfortable as hell. Being in her presence will bring to light every shadow, every part of yourself that isn't in integrity with your highest truth. If you have been running, numbing, avoiding yourself you will be completely triggered by the depths to which she loves and knows herself intimately. She unapologetically forces you to grow. What an incredible gift for humanity, to guide us home to ourselves, and collectively rise.

I stand beside the women whose stories are bound by this book, hand in hand, together, as we declare full reclamation of our power, and encourage you to reclaim yours.

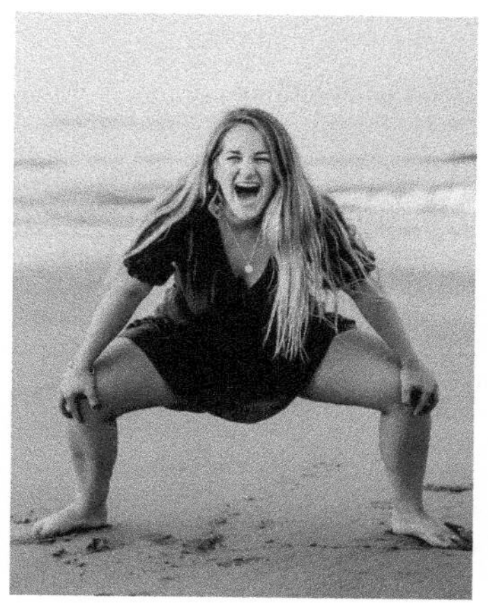

Amberlee Carney

Kia Ora, I'm Amberlee Rose, an advocate for women's empowerment, pleasure and sexual liberation. Among many things, I am an Erotic Maven, Pussy-Witch and Yoni Massage Practitioner based in Aotearoa.

My soul's calling is to work with women who are ready to move beyond the shackles and constraints of patriarchal conditioning, limiting beliefs and ancestral patterning; into a deep unshakable sense of truth, power and authenticity.

My passion is guiding women, like you, to become familiar with the inner realms of your divine feminine essence to awaken to your pleasure, power, creativity and that most rare and precious gift - your pussy.

I am wholeheartedly dedicated to facilitating and holding space for radical transformation, for you and myself alike - this work is my medicine and as women, we heal and rise together.

My offerings are Yoni Massage Therapy, Women's Circles, Online and in-person workshops and 1:1 Pleasure Awakening journeys. This is how I empower women with a better understanding of their sexuality, helping them to reclaim their bodies, sensuality and power in order to transform their lives.

I came across this work through my own healing journey from 13+ years of depression and anxiety - a major catalyst for a divine feminine awakening. I heard *her* call, I'd had enough, was tired of numbing out and was hungry for more from this life. This was a journey of learning to surrender all the ideas, beliefs, opinions and identities imposed on me to reveal and remember my true self, my voice, my truth and my personal desires. It was a journey of radical acceptance, deep self-love and sexual and personal liberation.

I continue to do this healing and transformative work for all women - to free us from the should's of societal conditioning, patriarchal oppression leading to perfectionism and burnout. To come home to ourselves, fully inhabit our bodies and learn to attune to the innate wisdom that spirals and moves within us. Deepen our connection to our intuition, sensuality, emotions, and our cyclical nature as women. Reconnect with our heart and wombs desires, creating stronger boundaries and clarity in decision making.

It takes a brave soul to step into this work, breaking social taboos, reclaiming your power to live your life guided by pussy. And if you are one of those souls, from my womb to yours, I welcome you home sister.

Instagram: @rose.revealed
Facebook: rose.revealed

The Shit Queen

Bec Cameron

I am beginning to write this chapter whilst I'm perched upon my porcelain throne. I am creating my 'zombie killer scent' as I spray my sweet A-grade, home grown, degradable, compostable, warm sloppy manure anywhere and everywhere! I'm glad this isn't the audio version ha! I am trying to blame the packet of Tim Tams I ate earlier in the day. However, *this* time there was also a sprinkling of reward - for cleaning the house in time for an inspection, specifically, the fact that I can see my bedroom floor for the first time in months. There's also a dash of self loathing, a hint of self sabotage, camouflaged with amnesia forgetting I would pay dearly for this choice of food and layers and layers of Trauma. Hello, nice to meet you I'm Bec … Oh wait let me wash my hands first.

I am a living, breathing, trauma recovery machine and so are you! By the end of this book you'll be reminded of how magnetically powerful you are. We are the same, yet each of us unique. A paradox, I know. The more I learn about trauma the more I see that we are all traumatised one way or another. I'm yet to meet someone who hasn't been traumatised, though I do believe anything is possible. I have been a walking advertisement for 'A PRODUCT OF TRAUMA' most of my life, it is only now that I am beginning to shed the identity I had as 'I'm a traumatised person' to questions of 'Who am I now?' 'How do I piece myself together?' 'Which old bits do I bring with me and which parts do I replace with new ones?' I have an incredible capacity for self-compassion alongside a deep dark pit of utter self-hatred. Fucken duality in all corners.

I want to share some of the traumas I've been through from my childhood, though it's an extremely difficult thing to speak of or write about. I hope I can convey them properly and do them justice. For much of my life I have tended to just skim over them, purely for the fact that there are so many and they're all quite equally heavy. The experience I've had when I've shared some of these is that most people can't even handle hearing them, and I can understand that to some degree. People don't want to believe awful things happen and the fact I'm relatively okay, most days, tends to make people feel maybe it wasn't as bad as what I'm saying. When I was younger, I would mistakenly tell anyone who would listen, just needing someone to hear me, help me or even save me. The outcome was them running away as fast as they could, which was most kids, or not believing me, which was most adults.

Even before I could walk, until the age of ten, I was physically abused by my father. Simultaneously from roughly three years old, that I know of, until ten years old, I was sexually abused by different individuals that were male and female. I saved myself from my father by stopping visits to his house on weekends. We left the church and that social circle at some point, which was where other sexual abusers had gained access to me. At my mother's house, when I turned ten, the last perpetrator didn't have as much access to the family as he once had, so I was able to hide from him. My mother knew all about the predators committing those acts of sexual abuse, she had even caught it happening a couple of times that I know of, yet she did not protect me. My extended family knew about the main sexual abuser as well, but did nothing.

All of that consumed me as a child and as a young adult. A lot has been blocked out thanks to my amazing brain and body for protecting me, however, if I do decide to think about it, I tend to remember something new each time. I try not to do that unless I'm in a strong place and am consciously willing. That's why when something triggers our trauma it can be so awful because we have no time to prepare ourselves. Early childhood trauma will affect *everything* from there onward. Our view of the world becomes warped in various ways. For me, I felt completely safe in dangerous situations, with dangerous people because healthy examples of what is 'safe' were never a part of my world. In my teens to early twenties I fought off multiple men trying to rape me; I was lucky there. In my early twenties I began dating men that were twice my age and I knew were dangerous; one of which became a murderer five years later. I lived in survival mode and as I grew older, started hating all human beings and seeing the world as a horrible dark place that I kept falling prey to. I was also attracted to the darkness of life, and even to this day I find pain and darkness so beautiful, however I now see it as my teacher and I know it is not my world any longer.

We see the world based on the experiences in our lives up to this very moment. As the saying goes, 'when we know better, we do better.' If all the people you meet in life are evil, you're going to think the world is only made up of evil. But how can you possibly tell yourself to hold onto hope, if you've never felt hope before? I'll tell you a little story about where I found hope for myself ...

I don't really remember what had led me to this point, I only remember the pain I was feeling. I was nine years old and my pain was relentless. I needed it to stop. I was exhausted, constantly terrified and I couldn't bear the thought of the rest of my life being that way. Even at school I was being bullied almost every day. I felt like there was nowhere I could be safe or find peace. One day I suddenly realised ... I needed to kill myself - that was the *only* solution for me. Even recalling that feeling of hopelessness now as I write this, brings up tears. Sadly, I truly felt it was the best option; kill myself or continue to endure the abuse for the rest of my life. At nine years of age, you have no foresight or any idea that life will change. I also had a knowing that I wouldn't be trapped here anymore, and that there was something better when we died.

As I began the process of killing myself, I was immediately CONSUMED and overwhelmed with a feeling I had never EVER felt before ... I had this sensation of comfort, of love, of knowing that somewhere out there, someone or some thing loved me unconditionally. It broke me down into a very sad and confused young girl. What the hell was this feeling? How can I feel love right now as I'm about to die? I thought, okay, can I pretend this is real? Let's try it. While looking to the stars at night from my bedroom window or scanning the globe in my imagination, I would think to myself, somewhere out there, something loves me, truly *truly* loves me. A week went by and I hadn't felt that beautiful feeling again and I was still stuck in my living nightmare. So, I tried it again. This time, the sensation came back even stronger than the first time. After that I knew it was real, and I decided to trust that feeling. I decided I would endure until I could escape. When the stars aligned, I was able to gather my strength. I began protecting myself, and lucky for me it wasn't much longer that I had to wait. When age ten came around, it was like everything fell into place and I could get some reprieve. The emotional abuse that followed in the following years from my mother, was far better than having to lose access to my body.

At age twenty and twenty-one, I had begun looking for answers about why we are here and what the fucking point of it all was. Why did I have to endure so much fucking pain already in my life? Where do we go when we fucking die? I started reading as many spiritual and religious books as I could. I also decided to welcome my psychic gifts back into my life. As a child I would see horrible demons and creatures, now knowing what I know, that would have been due to the environment and energy I was growing up in. I blocked them out and only allowed some of my psychic knowing to stay for my survival.

As I turned twenty-one many things happened. I see it now as an initiation from the universe. My first love broke my heart; I took my mother to family court to protect my baby sister; and I met the first person who got the ball rolling for me to start trusting humans. Her name is Belinda Pexton and she is a fucking force. I remember connecting with her at the bar of my first mine site job. I don't remember what our first conversations were, but she was very friendly. She would natter, she's a wonderful natterer, and she would speak about all these amazing things she's done or is doing, The next thing I knew I was on the bus going to her house for tea. I didn't even like tea at the time. When I got to her house some of my thoughts were, 'What the hell am I doing going to a strangers house?' 'You're leaving yourself really vulnerable, too vulnerable.' But slowly she showed me around and everything she had told me about herself was proving to be true. I could not understand this simple act of honesty. No one had ever wanted to talk to me without having some kind of agenda, or without lying about something. Even the boyfriend that had just broke my heart, cheated on me and told me to my face he never really loved me and just used me for sex. I took that incredibly personally; I know better now. Everyone I knew had hurt me and, I believed, anyone who hadn't soon would, or only hadn't because I didn't let them get close enough. After meeting Belinda, my whole foundation began to change. The way I saw the world began to crumble. She had my back. She was patient with me, gently guiding me to see things in new ways. She taught me to empower myself and began taking me under her wing as someone I could trust and who would be there for me. I never had anyone like that in my life before. I remember breaking down in tears while she was helping me paint the walls of my unit because I couldn't *believe* she actually showed up to help and was true to her word. We had spent a couple of years working together both in our place of work and in our friendship. She was helping me on my healing path and I was processing things incredibly fast with her help. She became a mentor to me. That was the start of my world changing. The start of realising the world wasn't all evil.

I remember coming across a book called "You Can Heal Your Life" by Louise Hay. At this stage I felt confident that I was a positive person and that I knew everything. Ha! This book showed me how negative I actually was within my mind. It gave me the starting point to changing the foundational beliefs I had about myself, that I wasn't a total piece of shit. This is a book I now buy for people. I always try to have a copy on hand to gift out. I try to re-read it once a year for a top-up and check-in with myself. As I began taking these baby steps into my healing I realised, with the help of kinesiology and Louise's book, that I hold all my shit within my body. The way I release it tends to be quite physical and literal hence the title of this chapter being The Shit Queen. Many of us hold so much emotional pain within our body. I let go of my emotional 'shit' by actually shitting. Some might even call it I.B.S but for me, when I'm in a very good place my shit is beautiful and I have no issues with my bowel, it even smells like roses. True story.

Prior to kinesiology I was trying to treat my bowels with a chiropractor. I remember one time she gave me an adjustment which caused me to have uncontrollable, explosive diarrhoea! Like if I needed to go it was coming out within moments!! I was trapped in the Pilbara for a week until I could get back to her to try click something else into place to make it stop. She did and I just went back to my normal constant diarrhoea. When I found kinesiology, it blew my mind and was an incredible blessing. Belinda had been trying to get me to go for 2 years. When I finally went for my session, I thought I was treating some mundane issues of people at work I didn't get along with. Well, that's what I thought I went there for. During the session my bowel issue came up and Teresa La Monica AKA Tess, the practitioner, treated it with an essential oil. Simply asking my body how many drops and how many times a day I needed to take it. After I left, it was like something magical had happened. Tess could pinpoint when big emotional events or traumas happened in my life to the year, month, week or day if I needed to know the specifics for my healing. This began a deep process of going into my subconscious mind to get the full story of my traumas, the extra shit you can't see or understand. Within two days of taking that oil I had normal poop. I asked her more questions about this and she said, 'we can treat your symptoms but in our sessions we work on the cause of the issues.'

I often have quite profound physical releases and they're all different. An example of one I had, happened 5 days after a session with Tess. I was walking at work and felt like I had hit my right calf with the boot on my left foot. As I took a few more steps my right calf felt very strange, so I lifted up my trouser leg to discover a huge bulging dark vein popping out through my skin. I got myself back to my boss, told him what happened and they had me out to the hospital pretty quickly. There I was then checked for deep vein thrombosis, but thankfully I was all clear. I searched up what all the symptoms meant in my 'You Can Heal Your Life' book as it has an added bonus of 'You Can Heal Your Body' book at the end. I looked up things like Blood, Right side of body and Veins. It was all related to the topics we had covered in our last session. Again, my mind was blown. I have many of these stories, even ones of non-stop shitting, literally until 5 minutes before I'm about to interview a powerful healer for my podcast, and then as soon as the interview is over, I'm back to non-stop shitting. Like the universe timed it so perfectly.

Throughout the years I have seen counsellors and psychologists, with no luck. Most just sat there with their mouths open, or told me how broken I was and were just not helpful at all. I felt some even did more damage. I can't remember how I heard about it, but I came across some information about Ayahuasca and long story short, I found myself sitting in my first ceremony not knowing anyone. The first night I ever drank Ayahuasca there was a part of the journey towards the end, where I felt that same unconditional love I had felt when I tried to kill myself. I realised, in that moment, this medicine had been calling me since I was nine, or maybe even my whole life. Thus, I began to cultivate a feeling of 'I'm not alone and I am loved.' It helped me to gain an even better understanding of myself and it instilled an incredible drive to plunge deeper into the self-healing aspect of my journey. On my search for healing tools, I didn't give up on the psychologist path and I now have a beautiful psychologist who understands me extremely well. The most important part, to me, is that she specialises in Trauma. She makes me feel safe with sharing my deepest and darkest thoughts. She makes sure I feel safe before I share any triggering stories with her, and she doesn't believe all the details are necessary. In fact, she feels it can be re-traumatising for us to go over the full details in some cases.

I now combine all the ways of healing I've found that work for me.

The thing I find most fascinating is how difficult it can be to change or expand our minds. I have been, and still am, lucky enough to have many people come in and out of my life, showing me different examples of what's possible in this life. Now I can't stop my own expansion and I will often go to bed with an aching prefrontal cortex when I feel like I am expanding my mind further once again, wrestling with a new concept or understanding a new perspective.

Growing your wings can be so fucking painful. Whilst inside of the cocoon, the darkness seems infinite. You then finally reach a point where you no longer wish to be in the darkness. You somehow find the strength to claw your way out, but as you struggle and fight to release yourself, you recognise your strength. Had you not gone through the struggle and process of emerging, your wings would not be strong enough to carry you. Owning your shit is extremely difficult for your ego to adjust to therefore, accepting your previous ways of being or thinking can be the hardest parts to shift. Believing anything is possible is a great place to find yourself, in regard to keeping your mind open. Slowly learning to accept the ugly parts of yourself, will grant you freedom in your daily moments of insecurity and loneliness.

I will leave you with this … Your story is important, and you matter! Sometimes you will have to be the one to remind yourself and you might be the only one that can, or will. Healing generally takes time and it can be fucken messy. It can also be subtle and very gentle if you can keep your heart open, looking for the signs. If you find yourself struggling longer than you thought acceptable, learn to accept that this is just where you are right now, and it could take you ten years to get through it, or it might be over tomorrow. If all else fails, run to nature. It will heal you, offer you answers and love you - all in the blossoming symphonies of the flowers and plants. It will bring you messages via the creatures that make their way to you. Look them up, learn about them, ask them to share their wisdom and thank them for assisting you. They protect us and serve us constantly.

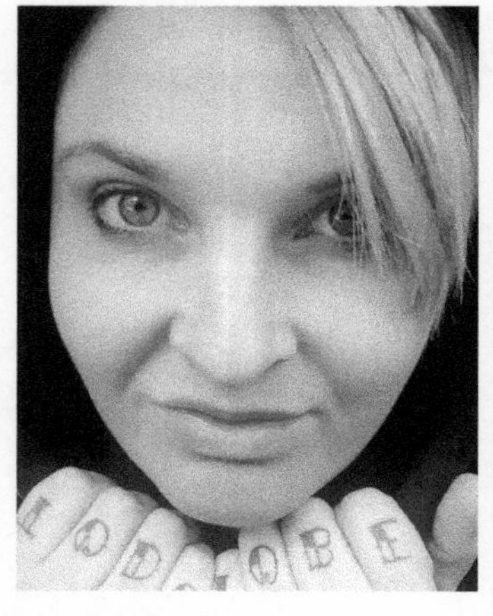

Bec Cameron

I sometimes have the illusion of being self-made, however deep down I know the truth. I stand upon the shoulders of every one of my ancestors who persevered, thrived and evolved into the wisdom keepers of my DNA. As we each heal ourselves, we heal all who came before us and all who come after us. We grow stronger together. I thank them for protecting and guiding each of us, whether we know it or not.

My name is Rebecca Cameron a.k.a Bec Cameron. I am the Host, Producer and Editor of The BeeSea Podcast. I interview and have conversations with some of the most fascinating people that I cross paths with. I endeavour to bring us all new possibilities - via conversation and to broaden our perspectives and healing at the same time. Podcasts help me personally so much and I thoroughly love learning about other peoples lives. I am amazed how they've overcome difficulties in their lives, how they see the world, how they lose and find themselves all over again.

I am also the founder of BeeSea Therapies which is located in Perth, Western Australia or online. There I work with individuals or small groups, creating safe spaces for healing and self enquiry to occur. I am honoured to be of service in this way and am consistently awe struck by the beauty of how spirit works its magic. I learn abundantly with each session and no two sessions are the same.

I was born with some psychic gifts and have been developing them further in my adult years. I have created workshops in order to teach others how to begin activating their own gifts, be them psychic or otherwise. I find everything incredibly fascinating when it comes to energy, death, space and frequencies. The limitless possibilities of life and what holds us all back. Our psychology, foundational beliefs and self-manipulation keep me bloody curious about the human condition.

I am also an artist, creating paintings, writing song lyrics, mixing amateur beats and singing. I dabble in photography and videography - just trying to have fun whilst adding more beauty into the world with the use of symbolic story.

I am looking forward to connecting with you!

www.beeseapod.com
Email: bec@beeseapod.com
Instagram: @beeseapod & @beeseatherapies
Facebook: beeseapod
Facebook: BeeSeaTherapies
Podcast: The BeeSea Podcast
(Find it everywhere)

Pathways

Bonnie Collins

One step at a time, that is how all of our stories evolve - how those steps feel and where they take us is the place to draw our focus. Some days we walk the path like a lightweight dance on the breeze floating down easy streets; other days we trudge an unforgiving and seemingly never-ending gauntlet. Then there are the days we cannot walk at all – stuck- still – immovable with the weight we carry.

So, with all the options, how is it that we come to choose the paths we step down? How do we take control of whether we are moving, dancing or trudging?

Is it a mindful choice, to knowingly and with purpose place one foot in front of the other, or do we mindlessly wander following others footsteps with no regard for our own direction? Is our path handed to us? Perhaps we are pushed and pulled down some paths, and once there given the choice as to how we next move, and how our stories are shaped?

I believe in life we experience a little of all these things, and as you grow your story becomes more aligned with whichever you choose more of.

Born into bodies that unapologetically take up space and take what they need without question – literally changing their environment to make it fit, not stopping to ask how we might impact those around us, traveling along our own path, it's instinct – its survival and it's what we do.

Somewhere along the way, we go from demanding our needs be met without question or apology, to shrinking our needs so that we are, in fact, minimising our own potential and existence.

At what point does that demand for ourselves stop? When do we choose to play small? What voice is it that has us believing we are not worthy of taking up space and having everything we need?

Perhaps it happens one little bit at a time as we settle into and accept the labels we are given. And this is a day one thing – we are born someone's daughter, sibling, niece, then we become someone's friend, classmate the list continues. Before we've even formed a grasp on our own thoughts, we've been taking on those of the people around us, when the time comes to ponder 'who we are' or 'who we want to be' and exercise our own choices, there is already a plethora of information to wade through. It can be easy to find yourself picking and choosing from other people's ideas and stitching together pieces you like (or they like), rather than growing into your own unique self.

That journey of growing up and discovering who you are, I believe, should be a path of selfish exploration, choosing should be a great joyful piecing together of the puzzle that is you, in your absolute truest form, coming to life with each little nuance that's sets you apart ~ finding your voice, your power and fully stepping into it.

For too many that is not the case.

For me, that time of being selfish, demanding I was seen and heard, ended before I could grasp its beginning. At 6 years old I found myself in a position where my needs were not a factor, and I was the one being taken from.

Being abused takes from you in a physical sense yes, but for me, no damage was greater than the words that were spoken to me, directly and indirectly by my abusers in their own attempt to keep their actions hidden, and as they talked amongst themselves, mocking to them, what were careless actions, but to me, was my very existence. The mental fuckery of not feeling like your physical safety was under threat (although they'd done that also) but warping and shifting truth and understanding, so that on one hand I thought I was special for being chosen, and then was blamed for their corrupt behaviour afterwards. That is what left a sea of confusion and shame that changed me in an instant, and continued to change me with each encounter and far beyond.

The bumping of heads, knocking of teeth, clumsy too small hands and laughter that I didn't understand as I was reduced to a method of practice, was bewildering and left such a sense of misplaced responsibility and complete emotional confusion. I remember living in fear, not of what these perpetrators would do, but of what would happen if people found out about it. Was I doing something wrong - not what they wanted? Would it make them feel bad? How much trouble was I causing? I took on the fault of these actions, staying quiet and puppet like in order to protect the perpetrators, my family, and me; to keep the peace and to avoid doing any more harm.

Along with the sense of responsibility I now carried for everyone else's feelings, I held onto shame because of how I looked physically; because I had "tempted my abusers by being friendly and beautiful." I was told everything happening was because of my own doing. And so the cycle began of believing I was the problem, that I deserved whatever happened to me and if people were upset by my discomfort, that too would be my failing.

It wasn't until years later, sitting in my classroom, hearing a talk on appropriate behaviour, what consent is and what abuse is, that I even understood abuse or realised I was a victim of it.

In my mind, the story had been told so often that I had corrupted these people, tempted them and lead them astray, it had become my truth and I carried the shame for what I had done to them and what this secret would do. This new revelation hit me with such force I lost all sense of self. I didn't know what was true in the world and what, or where, was safe. I had learned early that I couldn't be trusted and that my voice and presence would cause damage, so I had no concept of where to turn.

I had figured out how to bury emotions of all kinds very early on, mostly because I didn't understand them, and had been taught that there was no safe place to express myself, assuming there was something wrong with me. On reflection, I made cries for help in the form of sickness. I would try any and every physical ailment I could come up with in the hope that I'd be able to stay home and away from people or at the very least, someone would discover that something was wrong with me. But with this new realisation, emotions crashed in. Anger, rage, betrayal, disgust, confusion; they beat down on me like waves on a rock slowly wearing away the surface.

The truth came out eventually, or some variation of it, and in efforts to protect me from the fall out I was sent away while it was 'dealt with.' I understand why not having me around for the practicalities made sense and, in some ways, I was thankful to escape, but on another level, it still felt like removing me was removing part of the problem.

Adults in my life sat in a weird place of mistrust – would you hurt me or help me? I'd overhear conversations about me but not meant for me, which only gave me more conflicting information.

"That's just what boys do."

Was it?

Is it?

An exhausting line of questions and no answers played on repeat in my mind adding layers and layers of uncertainty.

My body and physical appearance became the enemy. Growing into a young woman seemingly innocent comments either said to me or directed at the adults in my life about me, all sounded so different, so distorted.

"You're going to be a real heart breaker." - WE KNOW YOU'LL DO DAMAGE.

"You better lock this one up." - YOU'RE GOING TO CAUSE MORE TROUBLE.

"She's very beautiful" - JUDGMENT NOT PRAISE – WE KNOW WHAT SHE'S GOOD FOR.

These comments screamed to me again that I would be doing something wrong and cause someone else harm.

So, I tried to hide. While my peers were entering the realms of teenage years excited and intrigued with the idea of dating and discovering, I was terrified of connection with people and of myself.

Having learned not to hear my own voice, let alone trust it, I only knew certain external truths I was handed. I was the skinny girl, the pretty girl, the nice quiet girl … and I hated that girl. I hated her body, I hated the attention she got, I hated how she moved amongst people, I hated desires I thought she was responsible for creating, and I wanted nothing more than to be anyone but, 'that girl'.

The path of self-loathing and punishment presented itself and I strode willingly along with no surprise that external 'truths' meant I eventually fixated on body image. I got to a stage where I stopped eating. Ironically enough I loved my food and I only stopped because I couldn't handle the attention I would get when people were surprised that I did eat. However, what really kicked this along for me was the sense of control I had over this one thing. It was intoxicating, and my frantic brain quickly clung to it, until I found myself a barely 40 kilo mess who simply didn't want to be here anymore.

My family and friends loved me and would tell me daily. They would tell me how worried they were, but no matter what they would say or how often I'd look in the mirror to try find sense in their concerns, I saw only what my mind projected, what it had come to believe. I saw a shell that I blamed for the life I had and was unhappy with, and I just didn't care.

I stumbled through most of my teens and early twenties, with a façade of trying to get my shit together. I was trying to eat more, working full-time, and I'd seen a counsellor and spoken about what happened. So now I should be ok, right? I was going to convince everyone, mostly myself, that I was fine – I could do this. The only way I knew how to operate safely was to be logical. I didn't want to feel out of control or vulnerable. I didn't want to FEEL at all. My need for control meant neither drugs nor alcohol were an option, so I lost myself in being busy. I would be the master of achieving.

Success on the outside worked. It looked good and was widely accepted. It made me seem 'normal,' ticking all the right societal boxes and the few people in my life that knew of my battles seemed happy to see that I was doing better, I was 'okay.'

The problem with putting together a nice story or presenting a certain exterior, is that eventually the cracks will show up. Real life creeps in with bouts of anxiety, poor sleep, burnout, returning to poor eating habits, and the biggest cracks were especially reserved for my relationships.

I had a one-sided, distorted idea of what I thought all men saw me as, and I had made it my quest to be something different. I wanted to prove that men could be my friends without wanting anything more from me. I was desperate for someone to validate that I was more than this body I was in, and had more to offer than just what pleasure could be taken from it. I wanted to be one of the boys, to not be viewed as female at all, and so I began to deny this side of myself, switching off my femininity as though it were something weak, and opting for a brash masculinity.

Really, I just yearned to be me, to be cared for, to feel safe enough to let down my guard. But that wasn't who people got to know, and certainly not who they entered into a relationship with. Inevitably relationships would fail because I wasn't being myself, and I was so worn down with achieving at life that I couldn't even do a good job of trying to hide it.

There were beautiful and meaningful connections along the way that I will cherish always, but I can tell you that meeting someone and loving them even to the very the best of your ability, when you don't truly love yourself, is a breeding ground for hardship and failure. The wounds you inflict on one another will be deep and long-lasting, and when eventually you can't 'make life work' even after ticking all the boxes, it's a very bitter pill to swallow that you are the one who has to do the work on yourself. To go back to the start and face everything felt grossly unfair, and even harder knowing there may never be any justice for the situation it all stemmed from.

I wish I could capture in my brain the exact moment in time the awareness shifted for me from being in life, to wanting and choosing to actually live it. If only there was one magical moment that we could selectively capture and carry out and, viola, the work is done. But there is honestly no such magic available, and this brings me back to how we step and move into our paths in life.

Sadly, and all too often it seems, it's never the easy paths that lead us to these moments. The pathways that birth something in you are the ones that leave you battered and bruised, and push you to new levels.

Obviously, this is only one of the many paths I've trodden, and it was not a path I chose for myself. It was a path I was led down, and the steps I was taking were clearly not my own, but along the way, there had come a point whether consciously or not, I made the choice to stay there and take up residence.

In the physical sense, I was no longer being abused, but mentally I had locked myself in the prison of that time and made it my home. I had become my own captor, my own abuser and I had learned the act well.

Realising and acknowledging this, I knew I needed to take responsibility for it and had to decide if I was going to keep going or to tear that path up and lay a new one. It's safe to say, the earthworks I knew would be required, were going to be extensive.

It is one thing to speak about something, to box it up and pack it away neatly somewhere so you can 'move on,' it is another thing entirely to let all the nasty sediment that has taken up residence in your very being, be stirred up, felt and released. And that is the only way through, otherwise we just add more layers, more hiding and more to unpack.

Emotional damage carries with it a very physical response and these beautifully human bodies that we dwell in are not designed to bury things down and carry that load. They will fight for you to show up as yourself even if you don't want to, even if you know you've been hiding, and when they can't fight they will fail, forcing you to take notice. You see the thing is, you bring yourself wherever you go, you cannot outrun yourself; you are made up of ALL the parts, ALL the steps.

So now, bit by bit, I would choose to reclaim all of me.

I learned to embrace the tears and anger and rage and sorrow; the cracking open of old wounds and grief for who I was, who I could have been, and what I had lost.

In this process I gained a new relationship, the most important I would ever enter into; a relationship with a small, broken untrusting girl who I knew could be anything she wanted to be. I just had to make her see it and believe it. After mistreating her for so many years, I would have to gain her trust.

I was in there somewhere.

No more masks

No more hiding

No more playing small

No surrendering my voice to pander to the comfort of others

No priding myself on my ability to be like a chameleon and blend in wherever I would go

No More

You will get all of me or none of me

She deserved that after all the years of hiding

I deserve that.

It meant getting uncomfortably honest with the people around me and being ok with letting go of things that no longer served me.

It meant saying no to continuing to be what I had always put forward, and accepting that my relationships would look different after.

It meant starting again and again as many times as required.

It meant turning the switch back on and feeling everything.

I chose to find my own justice. I decided that life mattered – that my future mattered – my existence mattered that I - FUCKING - MATTER and I chose not be a victim any longer.

Realising just how powerful my own voice is was paramount to my healing. I had, for years, let the words of my abusers take up space in mind. If simply repeating someone else's words that were untrue could have this impact on a life, what could speaking my own truth do?

Every day I would try out a new line:

"You are enough"

"You are loved"

"You are safe"

"You are valued"

Just one tiny truth at a time. More often than not, these statements would start out with the tone of a question and it was hard to persist in telling myself these things. We are often our own worst critics and give ourselves such conditional love.

On the days that were tougher than others to say the words and believe them, I would try to picture myself as that small child and think of how fiercely I would defend and protect my own child. I would try again with a gentler more encouraging and compassionate tone.

I chose to face things so I could be whole, so the people I loved would be able to love all of me back, and not be met with walls.

What started out as one tentative somewhat reluctant step towards myself, would grow to a walk, then a stride and now like an advance in battle, tearing towards myself as though my life depends on it – because it does.

Does that mean that I never falter? Never stop? No.

The difference is, now when I am presented with a fork in the road which could lead me down an old path, sometimes I coast right past without a second thought. Other times I will sit, not to wallow and dwell, but to acknowledge that the path also served a role in my making. There will be lessons deeper than I am willing, or able to learn at some stages, that I will be ready for in others. So I greet this part of myself like an old estranged friend. We don't need to jump back in as we were, but there are lessons available to learn from a now much safer distance.

I look at that girl, once scared of her own thoughts and being, and I see her write her own story. I see her look in the mirror thankful for the body she has, and all the ways it has served her. I see her not burdened by the thoughts of others. I watch her continue to make choices, knowing that good or bad, this is really being a part of it. It's messy; this life is beautifully fragile and that makes it all the more exciting to step right into it and FEEL.

I love this girl. This woman. Me

A woman stepping into her power takes responsibility for the choices made, which have delivered her to her current place. She may arrive seemingly late and little less polished than anticipated, but she knows the destination in which she stands is not a final resting place unless she chooses. With every step, life presents options for you to get to know yourself, to find the power you hold, to find your voice, to remember who you are, or to start again – choose to take them and then lean the fuck in.

CHOOSE

TAKE RESPONSIBILITY

FEEL

LOVE

And then TAKE THAT STEP

That is how we learn, how we heal, how we teach and how we pave the pathway for our daughters and theirs, to be able to dance more and trudge less.

The work will always be worth it.

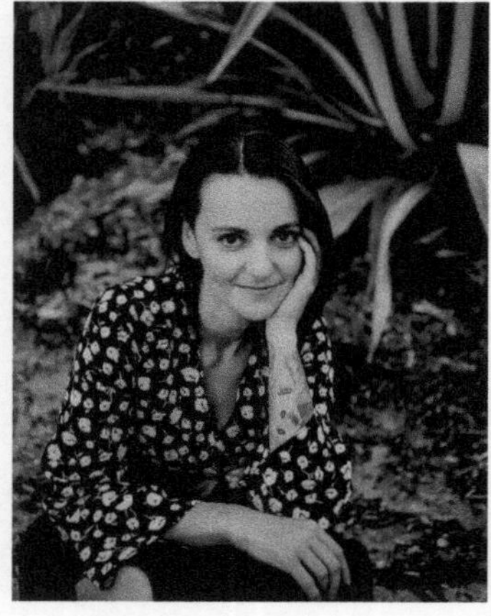

Bonnie Collins

Born and raised in Perth, WA, I grew up feeling disconnected from my own body, having worked for years on myself and with others I whole heartedly believe that the most important relationship you will have in your life is the one you have with yourself. The unison between the mind and body is designed to be a beautiful thing, and something I want everyone to experience.

I am an advocate for positive body image, self-love, positive thinking, doing the hard work and taking ownership of your own journey.

I also know this is not an easy journey and not one we are meant to do alone, so no matter where along the path you are I am happy to meet you there with a coffee, a word of encouragement and a way to bring you back into your body and stir up some energy.

I am a mother to one beautiful daughter and one of 8 children myself, so caring and nurturing others is a part of my nature. I have an honest no-nonsense and often no filter approach to life.

I found my ability to connect myself and others with their bodies through my love of movement and as a certified Pilates and Barre instructor I created "SWAI" a place for Movement, Health and Happiness. Offering a space where you are invited to be seen, to be heard and to be you – that is always enough. It's never about finding ways to change who you are but embracing all the different parts of you and building a relationship with each aspect so you can discover what makes you want to dance your way through your day and what has you looking in the mirror with nothing but pride and the excitement of what your tomorrow could hold.

www.swai.com.au
Email: bonnie@swai.com.au
Instagram: @swai_movement.health.happiness & @bon_collins
Facebook: bonnie.collins.9216 & movement.health.happiness

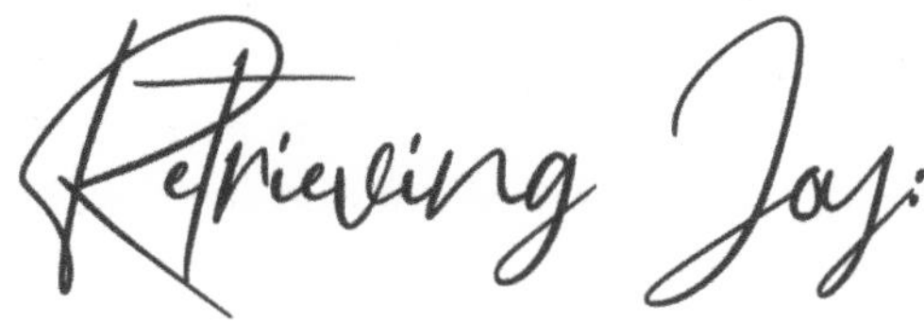

The Alchemy of Grief & Loss

Charlene Joy

'For every human being, the very first wound of the heart was at the site of the mother, the feminine. The Mother Wound isn't something we need to avoid or feel shame about. It's a doorway to our full power and potential.'
Bethany Webster, Discovering the Inner Mother

The dictionary defines *'Matriarch'* as a woman who is the head of a group or family. My interpretation of how the term applies to me is more complex. For a start, to be the chief, I would have to *belong* to a body of people. However, despite a lifetime of wonderful acquaintances and over seven sides of family, have I ever truly fitted in?

My broader families are filled with remarkable, generous, and outstanding humans. They are blessed with their own extended circle of kin to do life with. After the death of my mother and loss of connection to my father, I am no one's nearest or dearest beyond my home. My closest ties are to my beloved son and partner, both of which I am eternally grateful for.

I am not the boss of a marriage. Apparently, I am not the boss of my teenager. My brothers and sisters, somehow, have different mothers and fathers to me. I am the eldest of siblings and cousins, but I am no elder.

On social media, virtual friends share glamourous images connecting with chosen tribe. 'Forever grateful for our sisterhood. Our bond is beyond words,' they convey. Champagne glasses raised and adjoined; they celebrate the mysterious force pulling them together. The concept of soul family is alien to me. I could never grasp the *realness* of spiritual fellowship, either. Church, cult, or coven, I would feel like a total freak!

The Inner Matriarch

Being a 27/9 lifepath in numerology, INFJ personality, and a Yellow Planetary Seed sign on the 13 Moon calendar, I am born a mystic. Sun in Scorpio, Moon in Aquarius, Mercury in Scorpio, Pisces Rising… I am an old Soul, yet, I have been incredibly fragmented and 'split off' from parts of me.

'Joy' was the middle name of my Mum, who gave me the same middle name. I titled my chapter 'Retrieving Joy' because I had to 'go back' to reclaim Charlene. Denied and supressed, I had to welcome home and attune to the orphan within. To begin reparenting my inner child, I connected with my Inner Matriarch.

According to Heide Goettner-Abendroth, 'patriarchy' is translated as 'domination of the fathers,' while 'matriarchy' means 'in the beginning, the mothers.' Modern Matriarchal Studies puts an end to the prejudice that matriarchy means 'women rule.' It is true that in patriarchal societies women are ruled by men. But matriarchal societies are in no way the simple reversal of this scenario. In matriarchies, women are in the centre without ruling over other members of society. The aim is not to have power over others and over nature, but to nurture the natural, social, and cultural life based on mutual respect. Therefore, matriarchal societies based on a non-violent social structure, exist without the exploitation of humans, animals, or nature. Matriarchies have a social structure that values 'motherliness' in the broadest sense.

A wise woman has the inner wisdom of her mother, grandmother, and great grandmother, along with the wisdom of her own inner child. Corina Luna Dea suggests that, *'To end the numbness and shame that comes with not living authentically, we can find our way home by re-entering our story and giving meaning to the events that marked our life. We go back to the holy site and begin mining our memories… We have an opportunity to receive closure, forgive, grieve, and integrate pieces of our story into a new vision of ourselves.'*

Consistently mothering ourselves allows us to release the need to play small. When we mother the child within, we are cultivating an inner environment of safety and unconditional love. This heals the frozen energy of early trauma and brings our inner child into the present moment where joy and creativity can be brought into daily life.

What is one thing your inner child needs today?

Hiding Joy

When I would wag high school at 15, I would embark on my train and bus ride to Hyde Park. There I would enjoy a cigarette in solitude under the ancient trees, then wander over the road to the Theosophical Society. Thirsty for knowledge, their library was my oasis, covering everything from Alchemy to Zoroastrianism. Before long, high school kicked me out for never being there.

I was 16 when I enrolled in my first course on Self-Awareness. At 17, I told my grandfather I wanted to be a psychotherapist and study counselling. He advised me not to be ridiculous, 'I was too young!' Instead, I forked out tens of thousands on other courses in Naturopathy, Herbal Medicine, Reiki, Clairvoyance, Pleiadean Lightwork, and more. Some weekends I was nightclubbing, drinking, popping pills, being promiscuous and partying. Some weekends I was attending workshops such as The Turning Point.

As soon as I hit 20, I knew I wanted to keep growing. I moved from Western Australia to a *Fusion* training village in the mountains of Poatina, Tasmania. What began as a week-long 'Foundations' course, continued as a 6-month residential Certificate IV in Christian Youth & Community Work, then a 2-year Diploma in Youth & Community Work, specialising in radio, publishing, and youth outreach. During this formative time, I attended weekly Professional Integration Tutorials and my personal favourite, Group Life Laboratory weekends facilitated by Mal Garvin.

Around 30, I returned to Perth and joined a house church with a gorgeous bunch. I soon participated in a 'Relationships & You' weekend with MJB Seminars, which cracked open a layer of internalised shame I had not yet felt aware of. Then, found mentors in Sa and Claudio Silvano, Casey Terry, and Janet Bushby. Apart from revolutionary one-on-one work with Casey, I loved her 'trauma constellation' group processes, a spin on Hellinger's family systems. Casey invited me to begin her Integrated Trauma Healing Training involving Somatic Psychology, which I studied alongside my Bachelor of Counselling.

As I reflect on over 20 years of personal development, unique opportunities have paved my doorway to becoming a counsellor. The challenge for me will forever be deepening my recovery from post-traumatic stress. As a teen, I ignored my PTSD diagnosis and tried to heal my mind. Onboard my getaway train to 'self' development, I lost my WHOLE being. I intellectualised pain and wanted to save the world outside to avoid the world inside. To bury my wounding, I lived in survival mode, hiding my shame. No matter how many courses or books I fell in love with, I did not like Charlene. From multiple stressors in childhood, adolescence, even adult life, I have coped with complex trauma, perfectionism, body dysmorphia, depression and anxiety.

A while ago, I was privileged to be chatting with Darlene Lancer, author of *Codependency for Dummies* who proposed that I have had issues with emotional abandonment and codependency. I agree with Darlene. I have frequently felt stuck in my developmental trauma and projected my want for attachment onto others. Internally, I have reached out to others from my wounded child. Deep down, I have expected everyone to be my mother or father! Darlene's observation inspired me to further tend to my unmet core needs.

Killing Giants

I was 13 and Mum was given weeks to live, but she bravely persevered for 9 months. While I am devastated for her own unimaginable suffering, her dying birthed within me a lifetime of self-hatred and insecurity. My entire existence, shattered. As I welcome home my broken shards, particularly my neglected inner teen, I am no longer helpless. Furthermore, I am no longer invested in people who prove my deepest fear of me being worthy of rejection.

When Mum left her tumorous body, I felt a sick sense of relief by the permanency. The ambiguity of waking every morning not knowing if 'this was the day' was as terrifying as knowing she was terminal. When she was dying, I remember listening to the U2 song *With or Without You* and having an epiphany. Through Bono's lyrics, I recognised how I couldn't open my heart emotionally to be *with* Mum while she was alive, because I knew she was leaving. I couldn't live *without* her while she was gone, either.

This unsolvable scenario clouded my future lens and lingered in my nervous system, impacting my ability to connect healthily with others. Before becoming more attuned by being willing to step into the void, I super-imposed my unfulfilled wishes from early childhood and adolescence onto others. I struggled with anger and debilitating anxiety. When I confronted my fear and rage, they told me their real name: *Grief.*

Gabor Maté teaches that when we deny or bury our anger, it gets turned in against our body. If we shut down core emotions, which is a survival strategy, they could become a source of illness. How heartbreaking that when we suppress our sadness, or other 'negative' emotions, we inevitably suppress our Joy! There are consequences for acting out our emotions inappropriately, of course.

When we speak about our shadow, we often refer to the unwanted parts of ourselves such as jealousy, selfishness, guilt, or shame. The shadowy underworld is usually imagined as a dark repository for our fear of intimacy, unacknowledged narcissism, repressed anger, and unfelt sorrow. But Matt Licata, PhD, points out it is not only those aspects that we disavow and split off from. Many of us have lost the capacity to access and embody 'positive' states such as rest, contentment, pleasure, and creativity. In their nervous system, these sensations register as feeling unsafe. Some have disconnected from the simple sense of elation that comes from being alive!

Sarah Baldwin helps us understand integration by discussing how, when we experience trauma, different parts of us fragment or go into hiding. They run for cover (or they fight, freeze, or fawn) because there was not enough safety during the events that they were powerless in. As we enter our adult lives, these parts of us are left unresolved. They peek through our eyes now and see things like the past. When they perceive danger, they take over our system.

The behaviour that once helped was an ingenious adaptive response to survive but could become maladaptive when it persists to protect us from 'danger' that is no longer present. The 2017 fantasy drama, *I Kill Giants*, is a stunning illustration of how adverse childhood experiences cause fragments within. I could relate. Without ruining the story for you, the kid's movie left me with a profound mantra written by Joe Kelly:

'All things that live, die. This is why you must find joy in the living, while the time is yours, and not fear the end. To deny this is to deny life. To fear this... is to fear life. But to embrace this... Can you embrace this? You are stronger than you think.'

Braving the Void

To heal from childhood trauma, Dr. Arielle Schwartz considers it important to acknowledge the pain that you felt as a child. When you adopt a loving attitude toward the younger part of you, you evoke the same positive emotions that get generated in loving relationships between caring adults and children. Even if you didn't have a loving parent or caregiver, you can now create a reparative experience, which can help you find resolution.

Only months before my Mum and Dad's separation, we flew to Queensland for a family holiday. I was in Grade 5. Recently, I found a travel diary that Mum handwrote. On the day we boarded *Noah's Ark* to snorkel the Great Barrier Reef, she recorded, 'About half an hour into the trip, Charlene started vomiting and was sick for the remaining 2 hours of the boat ride to the reef, then for 2 and a half hours on the boat ride coming home.'

While I was in the water exploring, however, Mum described me being mesmerised and lured by the 'beautiful coral and coloured fish.' Nowadays, I crave the ocean, but will rarely snorkel due to a (rational!) phobia of sharks. The point I make is, that despite my hell ride to and from the reef, in the centre of my voyage, I struck gold. That rich turquoise and rainbow underworld was one of the most exquisite gifts. The bile in my hair was worth it! What captivated me even more was swimming near the edge of the continental shelf where the sea floor slopes into oblivion. From a young age, I could hear the mysterious call of the void. Would I find my *joie de vivre* in the *l'appel du vide?*

Everyone has inner gold. To discover it is our twenty-four-karat gift to ourselves. Matt Licata acknowledges our pathways of initiation and imagines a jewel being found within a weeping wound. He shares in his book, *A Healing Space,* 'In Vajrayana Buddhism, it is said that there is a particular quality of wisdom found in the core of specific difficult emotions, and the only way to mine that intelligence is through the direct apprehension and metabolisation of the underlying energy. If we prematurely 'go around' the emotion - repress it or act it out - or if we become flooded by or fused with it, we lose contact with that underlying wisdom at its core. Training ourselves to go into intense emotions; stay embodied with them; and infuse them with warmth, presence, and clear awareness is essential on the path of healing.'

The gold is not the trauma

The gold is not the trauma. Period. The gold is the healing. David Kessler explains how each person's grief is as unique as their fingerprint, but what everyone has in common, is that no matter how they grieve, they share a need for their grief to be witnessed. That doesn't mean needing someone to lessen it or reframe it for them. The need is for someone to be fully present to the magnitude of their loss without trying to point out the silver lining.

We ALL have grief, however much we delay, or bypass its expression. Robert Augustus Masters, PhD, suggests that grief works best when uninhibited. Many people want to muzzle or mute it, perhaps to minimise potential embarrassment. Anyone who wails, really lets it out, is often looked upon as behaving poorly or inconsiderately. Not surprisingly, Masters says, many of us end up in therapy to deal with grief that wasn't fully expressed.

Grief is the heartache, enormous hurt, and the deep opening. Unleashed grief is not mere venting or self-indulgence, but rather the undamming of our Life energy. Grief births a truer us in its wake. Masters writes, 'Where reactive sorrow contracts and isolates us, unimpeded grief expands and connects us, grounding us in natural openness.'

Joy is our birthright, but we cannot embody Joy if we keep turning away from our pain, trying to access the treasure without having faced the dragon. Joy is cultivating intimacy with our whole truth. How do we open in Joy? Masters describes, 'There's a sense of effortless expansion, as though our ribcage can no longer contain us. We radiate outward and usually upward, with not just our heart blooming wide, but also our belly, our throat, our face, our skull, our entire being. Joy lifts the sternum, opens the arms and eyes, lifts the head and step, loosens the jaw, and ultimately causes our body to soften and expand…'

Skilfully navigating the raw reality of who we are with our highs and lows keeps us plugged into Joy. When we turn to our original pain with the intention of processing our feelings, such as anger or grief, we retrieve our Joy.

Integrating Charlene

My high school English teacher, Mr. Sorenson, once gave me an assignment to write an autobiographical recount from my life. I decided to document the day my Mum died. It was therapeutic for me, but after I got my story back from being marked, I threw it in the bin (even though I received a high score!) Little did I know until years later, my grandparents salvaged my words from the garbage. Could I share my retrieved work with you? I was only 16 when I wrote it about the tragedy, which happened right after my 14th birthday. If triggering, please skip over or be sure to reach out to someone.

The cries of her pain still live with me. Do I follow them, or do they follow me? It was like watching someone being burned to death. If only water could have cured her misery. Her eyes rolled back as she threw herself around the bed in pure anguish. A twitch grasped the right side of her face. Her pleads for help were screamed in agony. The power of cancer governed her right to live as I, a useless spectator, prayed for her survival.

She was diagnosed with malignant melanoma. No cure. Cancer stole her health over nine months. Nine months of waiting to die. 'Everyone is living with the uncertainty of whether they will live to be one hundred years old or only one hundred days – my uncertainty is just more visible and obvious to others,' she whispered.

It was frightening to imagine a life without Mum. I could travel the world but never find her. I remember the first noticeable tumour. It was a small one on her stomach. 'Can I touch it?' I questioned as my hand reached for the grey bulge. I touched death. As time passed, that one multiplied into an entire body of observable lumps. Her bones were so fragile, she lost the ability to walk.

The final days left Mum in a comatose state. She laid on her back incapable of moving a muscle. I spoke. She listened. I gazed through her illness and found the beauty of a kind and loving face. A face that had always been there to guide me. The suffering she encountered was not deserved.

The day she passed on will exist with me forever. I woke with a feeling that her time had come. I got dressed for school. Perhaps if I ignored reality she would stay. I brushed my red hair for longer than it needed. Painted my face in colours of disguise. Only when I had dealt with the outside of me, could I tend to how I felt inside.

Mum was still breathing when I entered the room. Eyes shut, she rested on her bed while the cancer seized her body. 'Goodbye, my daughter,' Gran sobbed her heart out. I fixed my eyes on the woman who had once welcomed me into this world. Enthralled, I became drawn to her side. I was voiceless. Silence. In a feared place where nothing seemed to exist, I felt a warm hand turn cold.

A piece of me went missing. I only find her in my dreams. When I close my eyes, I can see her smile. If I listen carefully, I can hear her laugh. She loved me as much as anyone could possibly love their child. I have learnt how much I truly valued having a mother. I have learnt that it hurts when she is nowhere to be found. Tell your Mum how much you love her. When is it her time to leave?

Healing with Halinka Healy

Have you seen *The Shack* or read the book? I went to hire it from a shopping centre DVD kiosk, but it got stuck in the machine after my card was charged. An angelic matriarch with long, white hair stopped to help me. We had never met before. Halinka happened to be a counsellor, who had purchased numerous copies of *The Shack* on DVD for her clients. She instantly invited me to her home. We chatted for hours, then she gifted me one. The movie moved me profoundly and inspired my business, *Sarayu.*

Besides being a holy river in India, the Feminine meaning of 'Sarayu' is 'Flow.' The Masculine meaning is 'Breath of Life.' The 'ray' in my logo and 'Sarayu' portrays my infrared sauna service, offering radiant energy from sunshine. A divine ray exists in the human being, which shines with glory and gold.

Jules & Jewels

As soon as I decided to become a grief counsellor, I met Jules. I woke up from a hospital procedure and Jules was a patient in the bed next to mine. Another gentle, caring matriarch, she kept asking if I was okay. As our conversation unfolded, I was excited to hear that she had completed the same University degree as I was doing, on the same campus 20 years before me. A seasoned grief counsellor for people impacted by cancer, retired from years of service, I now get together with Jules for support when I need!

'Remember her as the day closes. You may have lived a life without an adoring, supportive mother, but if you look closely, maternal love has been faithfully beside you all the way. She was there for you in the stranger's kindness. She was in the wisdom of a caring friend. She was in the tender air of compassion when you needed it most. She was in your budding courage. She was in the mentors that guided you through the unknown. You learned how to trust your instincts from her teachings. She taught you about faith and of convictions and how to believe in your dearest of dreams. She is your spiritual mother, and she has been there for you in the hearts of many others – nurturing and caring for you, reaching you in ways only a mother's love can.'

Susan Frybort

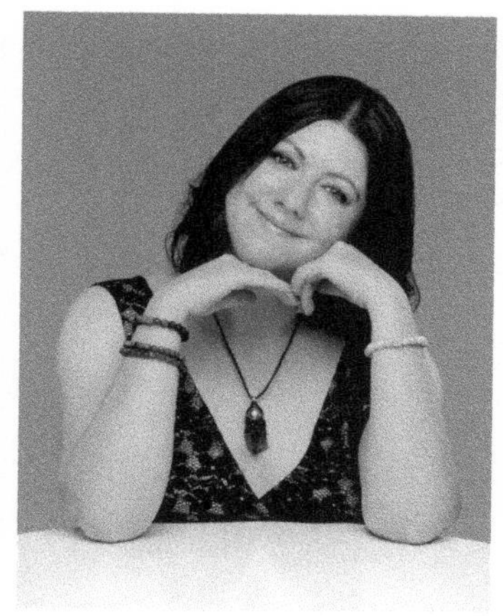

Charlene Joy

Hi, I'm Charlene Joy, Co-Founder of Sarayu Wild & Well in Western Australia where we offer a range of wellness & wilderness services, often existential & experiential in nature. We provide community events involving rite of passage, hikes for reconciliation, yarning circles, The Celestine Prophecy & Nonviolent Communication book clubs, as well as massage, low EMF infrared sauna detox sessions & more!

As I continue to grow in expertise as a Somatic Psychotherapist specialising in grief & trauma from a mind-body perspective, my approach is a synthesis of neuroscience, psychology & holistic practices in Eastern philosophy & polyvagal theory. With genuine capacity to hold deep liminal space for individuals, partners, parents, adolescents & children, I enjoy working with the ventral vagal complex of your autonomic nervous system. When you connect to your secure attachment biology within & with others, I believe you are free to express your real power & truth!

With my background in nutritional & environmental studies, I love to involve mitochondrial health & functional medicine. Educated at a University level & winner of The Gerty Ewen Scholarship in Counselling 2021 at The University of Notre Dame Australia, I create safety with profound compassion & radical acceptance. I meet you where you are, while providing a sanctuary for your joy & tears. Through shadow work & alchemy, Jungian & depth psychology, along with welcoming home your inner child & spiritual essence, I support you to be embodied & whole.

When you grieve, I walk *with* you into the void & valley of darkness, because I'm not afraid to journey there. I was 14 years young when my mother died from cancer of the sun. As I grew older, gold unearthed from my wounded core. Tears truly are seeds of joy! I found a divine spark within the smouldering ashes. I now help people transform their mysterious realm of psyche & soma into a blossoming, sacred garden.

Retrieve your joy with Sarayu Wild & Well events & services!

www.sarayuwell.com
Email: joy@sarayuwell.com
Instagram: @sarayuwell & @sarayuwild
Facebook: Sarayu Wild & Well @sarayuwell
LinkedIn: charlenejoy
Photo Credit: Image Style Studio

This Motherhood Mess

Emma Snelgar

I committed the cardinal sin while pregnant with my first child, in believing that my life wouldn't really change, and I would be the perfect mother and wife. I was quietly confident that it would all be great, and I would just *know* what to do. I would have the perfect sleeping baby who would considerately give me time during the day to cook, clean, read and do whatever else it was that I thought stay-at-home mums did. Our baby wouldn't affect our marriage, we would still be 'us', etc etc. Of course, it is indeed one of those things that you don't really know, until you do. But I thought years of shift work as a nurse, then a midwife, would prepare me for the all-nighters, and my experience as a midwife would count, when it came to actually living with a baby.

I worked hard to prepare for my birth and I am extremely grateful in that I had a beautiful waterbirth, and I rode that oxytocin high for weeks. This got me through the first few weeks of what turned out to be a lot of hard work to establish breastfeeding. Suddenly I realised why it was such an accomplishment to shower in the day, and that a tin of baked beans you can just grab and eat with one hand while breastfeeding, was a lifesaver.

My baby was a grade one clinger; did not want to be put down, ever. Showering was stressful, and he came to the toilet with me on numerous occasions. He thought 'feed/play/sleep' was a joke (more like feed/play/feed/feed/sleep/feed/sleep/feed/play) and 'drowsy but awake' was bullshit. He woke frequently, and only the boob would do to get him back to sleep. By the six-month mark he'd been waking five or six (or more) times a night, and was only napping for twenty minutes at a time unless he was on me. I was exhausted. At night, even when he was asleep, it would take me hours to get to sleep myself, just waiting for him to wake up again. His crying tore through me and my obsessive Googling had me convinced that the cry-it-out method wasn't for us. This, of course, caused all sorts of relationship strain, and as I was the one who was vehemently against leaving him to cry, I took on the brunt of his night waking's.

I bought this gadget and that book, looking for the silver bullet that was going to be the solution to his 'problem.' The sleep consultant I paid a ridiculous amount of money for, said breastfeeding to sleep was the problem, and I spent so many hours rocking and bum-patting that I spent longer being awake at each wake-up than I got to sleep in between. Convinced I was missing some key, some element that would magically make him sleep, I called Ngala, because surely it shouldn't be that hard. I must have sounded pretty desperate (which I was) as I got in to a day stay very quickly. As soon as we arrived, we were told it was nap-time and he was placed in a cold, sterile, unfamiliar cot, the door was shut and I was placed in front of the video camera to watch him 'protest.' There was no chat before-hand about what we had been doing, what he was like, what I was comfortable with. He cried and cried and cried. After a significant time, I was 'allowed' to go in and shush him, and eventually he cried himself to sleep. After his nap I was under-mined by the nurse. My concern about his sleep, and my own inability to sleep, were dismissed by both the nurse and the social worker. He was then placed in the cot again for his second nap, where he started to cry hysterically straight away. After a minute with my heart racing and adrenaline pumping through my body, I told them that I wasn't ok with this and we were leaving. I was told I obviously was 'not ready to make a change.' I don't know what I was expecting, but it wasn't that.

I was exhausted. I was having what I call the 'hospital fantasy' – where something happens to you that requires a hospital stay – a minor car accident (without my baby in the car, of course), or a kidney stone. (I have since had a kidney stone and I think this is still valid!) I would be thinking about the hospital fantasy whilst driving, and imagining how great it would be to have someone to take care of me, feed me and let me rest. Driving into a tree, not with thoughts of suicide but just so I could get a break, crossed my mind many times during this period. But of course, I always had my baby in the car and the thought of anyone taking care of him but me always brought the fantasy to an abrupt halt. He wouldn't take a bottle, didn't settle easily for my husband, and the thought of him crying for me and me not being there, made me feel sick.

I went to a GP because, although I was so incredibly tired, I couldn't sleep. I told him how my baby woke up every two hours or more, but even when he was sleeping I would lie awake for hours, my brain buzzing. When he woke, I could feel adrenaline surges running up my back. I had been getting three to four hours of sleep in twenty-four hours. I walked in on the verge of tears, and the fucking GP just looked awkward. He prescribed me temazepam, and suggested

I leave my baby to cry. That was it. In hindsight I was very clearly displaying signs of post-natal anxiety, yet despite me coming in with a pretty major red flag, I was not screened (I was also not screened at Ngala). I didn't bother going back or trying another GP.

The thing is, I could have easily fit into the category of PND and PNA, but I didn't feel like this was entirely true for me. It was entirely situational, based on my extreme, prolonged sleep deprivation. Every now and then my husband would hint that he was worried about me, but I shut him down pretty quickly. I knew it wasn't depression, but I didn't know what it *was*. I had no issues connecting with my baby, and I still enjoyed doing 'things,' though I found my 'things' had changed. It wasn't until I came across the work of Dr. Oscar Serrellach years later where he wrote about, what he coined, post-natal depletion, and it all started to make sense. Tired and wired, no reserves, running off adrenaline and cortisol, well fuck; that was me. I was depleted, and the depletion enhanced my anxiety, which I never really noticed prior to having my baby.

I had also fallen into the 'Mummy Martyr' trap, putting myself last and not speaking up to ask for help, because having to explain what you needed was harder than just doing it yourself. So I just got on with it, self-silencing myself. To quote another expert in the field, Amy Taylor-Kabbaz – 'we don't get mad, we get perfect.' I hid my struggle so well, because what was the point? There was no-one who could fucking help me anyway., My baby really only wanted me and having 'help' from anyone else came in the form of looking after the baby, which often made him cranky if the help lasted longer than twenty minutes. What I really needed was someone to help look after ME. Not just a nap here or there, but a week (or more!) of solid rest. And because I was so tired, I couldn't think clearly and was making stupid mistakes. I had to go to the shops multiple times a week because I couldn't plan more than a day or two in advance of what to cook for dinner (and I was so determined to 'do it all' that I didn't ask for help - like a dickhead). I backed right into a parked car with the reverse sensors absolutely screaming at me and I didn't even hear it. I even left the house with the front door wide open (multiple times). I really must have some pretty magical angels watching over me because I am so bloody lucky nothing truly bad happened!!

The thing I really struggled with was, '*why was I finding this so fucking hard*?' I was going to be the perfect mother!! Yes, I was tired, exhausted, but now *everything* was hard! I was exactly where I wanted to be; I loved my baby more than anything, I loved being his mum and looking after him, I loved my husband, but I often felt stuck. I missed being able to just walk out of the door with my keys and handbag. I missed just getting up in the morning and having a lazy coffee or two without interruptions, or staying up late to watch a movie without having an anxiety spin thinking about the lost sleep I probably wouldn't have had anyway because I couldn't actually fucking sleep! And the guilt of feeling this way made everything feel even worse. I was going through Matrescence; the term which characterises the transition from Maiden to Mother (much like the process of adolescence from child to adult). Like in adolescence, there are highs and lows, great moments and really shitty, awkward phases. You are reconciling your expectations ('sleeping like a baby') with the realities ('please oh dear God will you just go the fuck to sleep') of motherhood, whilst dealing with the feelings and responsibilities of your new role as a mother and simultaneously grieving for the easiness of your old life. You can't believe you ever considered yourself to be tired pre-kids. Old wounds from your upbringing might also emerge and need to be dealt with, friendships and relationships will change, and all this goes on along with the ridiculous mental load of health checks, shopping/cooking, washing, cleaning etc. With all this going through my head, throwing in insomnia and extreme sleep deprivation for funsies, its no wonder my brain felt like it resembled a dropped pie.

Was it this hard for everyone? Why was no one talking about this? Are we all so entrenched in maintaining the 'perfect mother' façade? The struggles of life with a baby are not spoken of, and if you find it hard, then 'you clearly aren't doing a very good job.' Mums have become forgotten and overlooked; our 'village' is non-existent. And whilst we are in the thick of it, we are too tired and overwhelmed to be coherent, or articulate advocates for ourselves, and life becomes reactionary instead of being proactive. We are also having babies later in life, and with this, comes new challenges. We have often already studied, learnt a trade, and been an active member of the work force and wider community, which has all become a big part of our identity. We are used to being in control, knowing what to expect each day, have our appointments scheduled, having a set lunch break, having an income. Our mums, if they live nearby, often still work full-time. The only preparation most of us have is four lots of two-hour antenatal classes which don't prepare you for what to do with a baby once you get home and the midwife and child health nurse visits end. There are so many different opinions and conflicting advice (which is mostly not based on actual science), that it can drown out our own inner voice, our instinct. In fact, so much of the advice out there actively encourages you to ignore your instinct. The day I told Ngala to fuck off and picked up my crying baby, was the day I started to take some of my own power back. (I want to add here that this is not to shame anyone who did sleep-train, at all. This was just not the right move for me, my baby, or my anxiety).

But I still had no idea what the fuck to do. I still couldn't sleep at night, my baby still wouldn't nap for longer than twenty to thirty minutes at a time during the day and he still woke two-hourly or more overnight. Not long after my disastrous Ngala visit, my mum dropped by one morning before work with a container of soup. I opened the door and completely broke down. She called in sick to work and sent me back to bed. She developed a plan that for the foreseeable future, she would come past in the morning from about 7-8.30am and look after my baby so I could stay in bed, and she would bring him in to me for his first nap and we would co-nap. She did it with no hesitation, and she did it for six weeks. I never would have even thought to ask, thinking that I had to get through it by myself, ever the mummy-martyr. But this was a big lesson for me, I didn't have to do it all by myself. I didn't have to be the 'perfect mother,' in fact, the 'perfect mother' doesn't exist. People wanted to help. Of course, not all offers of help are actually helpful, but as he got older I found it easier to rely upon and trust other people with him as well. I am just really, really lucky that my mum lived close by, was amazing support, and could be flexible with her work arrangements.

And so my long journey to recovery began. My baby wanted me close to him to sleep, and I surrendered. For every nap, and through the night. We started co-napping and co-sleeping from there on. He slept for longer, and although I couldn't always sleep, still, I was resting. I went to see a naturopath who diagnosed me with adrenal fatigue and put me on all sorts of supplements. I still couldn't sleep at night but I felt better during the day.

I didn't love co-sleeping all the time. It often felt like having an eight-limbed gremlin hanging off my nipple for most of the night. but it worked. By not putting the energy into the fight, I was able to conserve it to heal. By surrendering, and learning to block out all the white noise of other people's 'should,' and instead by focusing on what worked for me and my baby and what would get us through this trying time, we found some peace. I found support online from Facebook groups that supported people who also embraced co-sleeping, babywearing and breastfeeding, which helped immensely. This helped me to feel less alone and 'alternative,' and helped me to navigate my way through other challenges that arose. I still had wicked insomnia, but eventually found my way to a kinesiologist who used voodoo and magic, and my sleep did improve. Once I could actually get my brain to switch off, it was a matter of rolling over and switching boobs and going back to sleep - no more staring at the ceiling for hours on end.

My husband, of course, was not a fan of it. At. All. As much as I am fond of the man, he can be very 'conventional.' But the further I went down the rabbit-hole of sleep deprivation the less I found that I cared about what others thought (quite frankly I didn't have the energy to care!). As I slowly recovered from being the zombie-monster, and had become to bearing some semblance of myself again, he began to accept that it was necessary. He even co-slept with my eldest for a number of years when I slept with our second baby in the spare room! (They really can change, a large reason why I love him so much!)

The thing about motherhood is that it does, in one way or another, break you. It will tear you down until you are just a kernel of your former self. But the beauty is that of course, nothing lasts and you do get to build yourself back up. You can pick and choose which parts you keep and which parts you just leave behind. We might keep the 'work appropriate' mask, but leave the part behind that tolerates misogynistic bullshit at family events, because who has time for that anymore anyway. You might start thinking differently about the planet and how you care for it now you have the next generation of caretakers literally right in front of your face. You will be forced to come face to face with your own inner child and you will reflect on how you were parented. You may make choices that are different, and you will have to be ok with that choice causing upset. This place is from where I started to grow and nurture my inner Matriarch. I grew and evolved, and unapologetically parented in a way that felt right and natural for me and my babies. And I will fight for them every day of the week, no matter who I upset along the way. Because it's not just about me, and it's not just about them: it's about us, together. And although my husband and I have had our differences, we have grown together and evolved into a cohesive family unit. We weren't always on the same page and that was sometimes hard and incredibly frustrating for both of us. I imagine it was hard for him to watch me slowly lose my mind! He respects my choices, my instinct, and my inner Matriarch, and I am grateful that we have come through stronger.

I was lucky I was able to find the help when I needed it most, and I am aware that there are so many others out there who are mothering without their own mums (or maternal figures) nearby. Husbands are great, but they are not a replacement for the proverbial village. It had me thinking, how can we fix this? How can we make motherhood be valued again? I have dreams and visions of what we can do to change this, and I have started studying different courses as the first step, because no mum should think that driving into a tree or getting a kidney stone sounds like a great way to get a break.

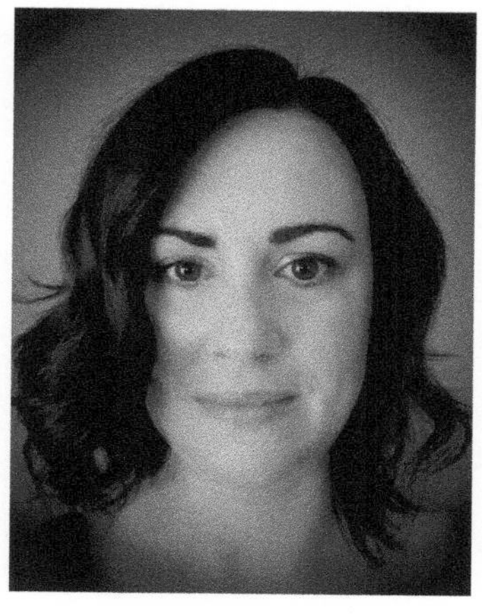

Emma Snelgar

I've always been interested in babies - for my first ever 'assignment' in year three I chose to write about foetal development from conception to birth. After high school I studied nursing knowing that midwifery would ultimately be my goal, and I always knew that somewhere in between I would have babies of my own.

Midwifery however turned out to not be my final destination as I found it difficult to work within the hospital system that is essentially set up to dis-empower women. As soon as I handed in my resignation, I found a research job within the Telethon Kids Institute where I get to see mothers and their babies in my clinic every day, and it is important work that I am extremely proud to be a part of.

Working with mothers and babies has turned into my passion and all these different experiences throughout my career, as well as my own personal journey with motherhood and what I have witnessed my friends go through, have brought me to where I am now and I believe that this is where I meant to be. There is a serious lack of support for women in the system after they have children and I want to do what I can to help change that. I have completed the Mama Rising Facilitator program with Amy Taylor-Kabbaz, a leader in the field of matrescence so I can help guide other mothers through their own transformation into motherhood.

I have also started a certificate in Applied Mental Health Studies with a focus on Perinatal and Infant Mental Health, which will lead to a master's degree. I want to change the system – from the way that pregnant women are educated to the way that they are supported after baby is born, and this is just the first step.

I have two very funny, happy boys who now both sleep all night (it eventually does happen!) and a wonderfully supportive husband. I am a voracious reader of mostly fantasy and fluff – I'd much rather be reading than doing most things, and I love listening to feminist or personal growth podcasts while I lie next to me wriggling youngest while he goes to sleep each night.

www.empowermatrescence.com
Instagram: @empowermatrescence
Facebook: EmmaSnelgar

Bullied

Gezzell Sabina

So I was bullied … for blowing my nose too loud. Yep you read that right … So you know what I did? I blew it as loud as I could. And this became the awkward path that I chose. Have you ever felt like you're breathing through a straw while looking up through murky, black water, hoping no one treads on your face or you'll stop breathing? Well I have felt like that more times than I would like to say, but each time I couldn't find my way out, or catch my breath, there was always something stirring in my soul that told me to keep going. Pick your tits up, as a friend once told me. And so I did, every time.

It wasn't the easiest growing up for me, far be it violent or dark. I actually come from a loving home. Struggling though, internally. I have always been told that I'm the black sheep, or the odd one out, round peg in a square hole, you name it, I've felt out of place most of my life. Within family circles, at school, and friend groups, but epically when I was younger, no matter what, there was always a big part of me that was content and secure just being me. What an oxymoron hey! Somehow I always knew my soul was different, stronger and yet so very fragile for a reason. I mean you don't get given a name like Gezzell Sabina Cox and not have much to say. Being the youngest in my family didn't always have the best benefits; I am ten years younger than my brother and eight years younger than my sister, so that's a generation gap right there. My brother and sister had each other and I kind of didn't have anybody except myself. There is a positive spin on this though, I had a brother and sister but once they left home, it was like being an only child.

The problem with feeling like an only child was having to deal with things alone, and for me my darkest times were during high school, a long time ago now, but this shaped and scarred my life. School can be tough at the best of times but when you are a bucked-tooth, tall, pimply easy target, with a name that reminds hormone jack-up assholes of cum, well, high school was just fucking shit.

For all the darkness that the prestigious high school that I went too had, I am glad that I suffered it out and didn't actually have a '13 reasons why' tragedy. Always trying to understand what 'they didn't like about me,' why I didn't fit in, and why I was the brunt of so many jokes. There were years of hurt and pain. But this one day, (no not at band camp) I was about fourteen or fifteen, I still remember it so clearly, my mum had taken me to our beautician, (I wasn't allowed to shave, only wax. Talk about another layer of pain for a teenager; the physical and then just another thing for the kids to pick on me for pffffft) and she was one of those 'beacons of light' kind of people. She said to me that when she was walking through a shopping centre she would smile at people. One day an older gentleman stopped her and thanked her for the gift she gave him. Confused, as she didn't know what he meant, he said 'your smile is like that of an angel and you have brightened my day and lightened my heart.' From that story and the recognition of the amazingness of inner beauty in my own soul, that was the first time (of many) I took my power back. I had always wanted to give to others, be a people-pleaser even when they were being assholes, but from then on, I actually saw the beauty in being beautiful. The last two years of high school were different for me; the bullies still kept trying to get a bite out of me, and sometimes they would, but most of the time I found some internal power and got through.

This was the start of remembering to always come back to self, and it can be very hard to tell the story of yourself, there are often so many stories to tell. I was brought up not to be vain, 'Children should be seen and not heard.' I'm not sure how many times I heard that as a child but it is one that stuck with me, and it really does suck. We all have a voice and should never be told to quieten it. So even though I tried, and was (and proudly still am) the loud one, the noisy one, the one who swears like a truck full of troopers, being loud can make it harder to fit in. Being loud, though, enabled me to feel like I had a purpose. If I could get a laugh, or a shock reaction out of someone then I could give them the chance to feel something different to what they were feeling before.

So that was the basis of my teenage years, the years that shape who and what one becomes – apparently …

I grew up with no real hierarchy of older women guiding me, for the most part it was just my mum and I. There were no really close aunties, cousins, or grandparents that lived close enough by to go to for advice and guidance, so I was forever searching for something bigger, pretty much alone. Always pulled towards the earth and Wicca, I was too afraid to really commit to being and practicing as a witch. The constant internal battle of wanting to believe what I was feeling when I thought I was using magic, and the scientific side of my brain telling me 'you need proof,' was forever my challenge. I had such a deep calling to trees, plants, herbs and natural medicine; that's where I found my calm. And, as time went on my tribe people. But being the people-pleaser with that underlying desire to fit in and belong, my ability to know who to let in, was not a strong point of my character. People are innocent until proven guilty, Right? This didn't always work in my favour. Being generous with my energy allowed for a lot of broken shards of my heart to fall and be given away and the loss of my goddess power, given to the wrong people. But no matter the darker hurting hearts, I would always find some beautiful diamonds.

Now we fast-forward a few years (there are many stories to fill in this gap but that's for another time), to where being an adult I had, (or so I thought) a grip on bullying (yippee win for me for a little while). Finding what I thought was my calling as a healer through remedial massage and laying hands, was so fulfilling, but there was always a yearning, something that I wanted more than to just help people heal. I then faced one of my hardest, but most rewarding hurdles; I became a mum. But this wasn't a smooth easy transition for me and my body gave out on me more than once. It's such a roller coaster of emotions and that transition of I want to be … Wholly shit, what if I am? … OMG I am … No sorry now you're not!

Falling pregnant was the easy part for me, keeping them was not. When I was twenty-three, my then partner (my husband now) and I fell pregnant, when we were six months into our very fresh and passionate relationship. I had just bought my first house, he was on a 4 & 2 FIFO (Fly in fly out miner) roster. Oh and did I mention he was four years younger than me. So a ripe nineteen year old and a twenty-three year old, great job, great new relationship, and mortgage. We just didn't think we were ready for that HUGE step. So we, I say we but really it was me, decided to have a termination. It still breaks my heart to this day that I didn't keep her, as she was the only girl that was to come through. I know that 'they' say that you don't pay the price for things such as this, but fuck me I did … Lesson after lesson after lesson - I lost three more babies after that termination. I paid my dues. And I hope she can feel me and I hope she knows how sorry I truly am. One of our losses ended up in an ectopic pregnancy where I had to have surgery had one of my tubes removed. Guess what side? Yep the left tube, my feminine side. After the ectopic, there was one more miscarriage that we were both really present for. After seeing the ultra-sound and being told all looked good, we were happy. I felt off one day so had a shower, he jumped in with me, and there I bled out another child that could have been ours. I cried, I was hurt, I was so fucking sick of 'paying the price' that I actually surrendered and gave in. All the hurt I had carried for the little ones I would never hold flooded out of me, and this was the best thing I could have done. From there, I actually allowed my own healing to take place. I found I had to stop playing the victim; yes this happened to me and yes there were things that I could have changed or done differently, but a friend at the time said to me that Mother Nature/Gaia only gives us what is needed for both souls to fulfill their soul path. I found the strength to forgive my body; for not doing what she couldn't, my soul for not being ready, my heart space for needing to go through these lessons. I had never really done any manifestation work before and by goddess I was ready to try again when I was about twenty-seven, (Saturn return right lol). So I pictured my belly growing, the beautiful golden diamond of light that was my womb space being the best place for my baby to not only come into, but to stay. and be loved and nourished. It was Easter 2008 and we were away camping. I turned to my partner and said, 'right lets go to bed babe, we are going to make a baby hehe.' The next morning I knew that my glorious son had come through and this time he was staying. So at twenty-nine, I finally became a Mum.

I have two beautiful, loud (wonder where they get that from), very active boys. And the next phase of bullying reared its head. My first cautious born, with the most gentle and fun loving soul, had a hard time with schooling with his reading and writing, so much so that the school he was attending told me I needed to get outside help. Like we weren't paying enough in school fees that we needed to outsource tutoring and pay for that as well. My other boisterous boy, well he would give Evel Knievel a run for his money; always on the go and forever doing dangerous, 'stoopid' boy things. Most of my mum friends with boys got it, but friends who have only girls, or nice quiet subdued boys, have no idea what it's like to have a firecracker for a kid. As the boys got older and with the push, more like shove, of school, friends, and fellow parents, we had the boys tested and they were both diagnosed with ADHD. My eldest one has inattentive ADHD, so he has a hard time focusing on one task at a time, and my youngest has ADD with energy to burn, and an attitude to boot.

So here was and still is, the next big challenge I faced with not fitting in. And I can tell you that thirty years on, kids and adults can still be so cruel. And as an adult I now know that it's more from the environment that a person is in that shapes their opinion on the rights/wrongs of society. My boys know they are different, the constant looks and things said about them make it hard from them not to be aware, but they chose me to help guide them through. One of the biggest struggles coming to terms with the boy's diagnosis was whether we medicate them or not. Wow, did this trigger all sorts of failures in me as a mum. As a mum who always tried to be so natural with their diet, immune boosting system, sporting activities etc., the thought of putting them on medication just made me cry. A lot. With drug addiction on both sides of our families, the fear that this would open all sorts of cans of worms was too much to bear. I found myself living on the river for a while (De Nile that is!), and believed I could 'make them better.' How foolish I was. But after getting over my own victim, failure mum moment, I did some research and took them to a paediatrician where I finally understood that this was not a fixable situation, but something that can be managed. With help and knowledge, we can work together to give them the best tools for them to be happy and confident. So yes, we did put the boys on medication. This is still a hard thing for me to accept, and I hope that I have made the right decision. But at the end of the day they are my boys and I will do what I feel is right for them. I am not a backseat mum, I turn up, I am present, I give them what I can, I do this so that they will be fabulous men one day and know that they have the ability to be and choose what they want to be. I will make sure they are good people. And isn't that what most of us want for our children; they need to be able to be them. And for those who can't understand or in most cases of the people I have come across don't want to understand, I need to do what is right for my boys. They have chosen these challenges and blessings for their lessons. The hardest lesson my soul wants to learn, is acceptance. I have been through lesson after lesson and for the most part have done alright. I am honoured that my boys chose me, even when I am forever pulling my, now greying, hair out.

As a soul having a human experience, and with my love for the unique, I am here to not only learn for myself, but to teach my boys, and hopefully their friends, the different and the magical wisdom that comes from our Mother Earth/Gaia and the cosmos above us. This has always been something that I have felt I belonged to. Even as a child, rocks, crystals, the stars, our great givers of energy from the trees, always had a way of comforting me. I am an energy giver, I feel best when I am making people/souls feel at peace, understood and loved. This is my alignment to my higher self and the true essence of my being. I am a facilitator of the healer inside the hearts of those who are searching for healing. I don't believe that any one person can be 'just a healer.' I believe we have the tools inside of us to heal ourselves and our past, but only when we have surrendered to the darkness that can plague us. I have lived by the saying 'the teacher will surface when the student is ready,' for we are forever a teacher and a student of time and lessons. I know that all the trials I have chosen to go through allow me to feel connected to not only my boys, but my family, friends and even strangers. The darkness that we can sometimes find ourselves in gives a great opportunity, if you allow it, to reflect and grow. I look back at my hurtful time in high school with a fondness that I got through it with a strength of character that allowed me to be the loud nose-blowing, foul-mouthed, fabulous, strong woman that I am now. I know that I have a huge empathetic heart and this is my gift to the world. I am so excited to see where all of my boundary pushing will lead me and the healings I can assist with in the future. I am grateful for the lessons that are yet to be had and the strength that I have found to move through anything that can come my way.

I am about to enter the next chapter of my life with tweenaged boys. And as freaked out about this as I am, I have faith that with the foundations I have laid for us all, we have the ability to be a powerhouse of awesomeness. This isn't to say that there won't be struggles and heartache, I'm sure there will be, but we will be ok. Knowing what my true essence is, and longing for justice in this world, I can say that I won't stop learning and growing, trying to always be there for the next person that may need a little Gezzell energy to keep going. I believe this whole heartedly for we all come from the same source. One of pure love.

So, even though life can suck sometimes, like really suck … big fat hairy balls …if this book has found you, and you are reading the amazingness of the powerhouse of women gathered here, you know that life is and can be fucking amazing. No matter what happened to you, the good, the bad the downright ugly, YOU have the ability to change your now moment. That is, if you choose to!

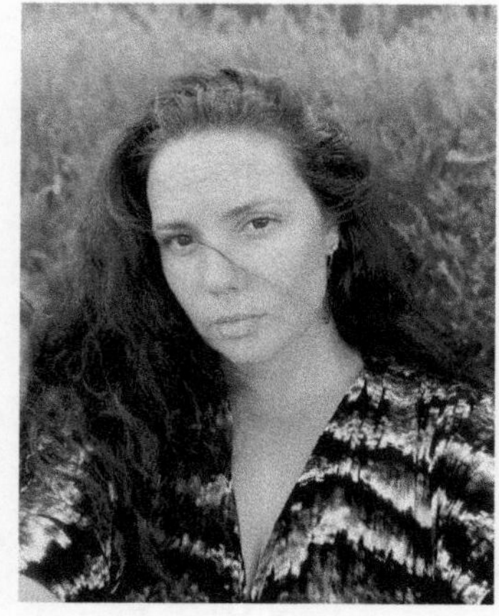

Gezzell Sabina

Hi, I'm Gezzell, loud, somewhat opinionated but always willing to not just listen but hear others viewpoints, what you see is what you get woman.

I lead with my emotions and wear my heart on my sleeve, offering a piece of it to those in need. Like the Queen of Pentacles in the Tarot, I am the maker of my space and love to open my home to nurture not only your soul but your tummies. I love to give I find nothing better than being a safe place for family, friends and clients to find sanctuary if only for a moment in time.

I am at my best when I am called into the healing vibrations of others ready to help themselves. With a background of nearly 25 years of massage therapy healings, I offer, to the best of my ability, natural healing suggestions for one's body, mind and soul. Touch is a powerful tool and a hug from even a stranger can heal so much. I adore giving hugs and believe in the healing that it can give.

I feel very strongly that we are all here for soul lessons, to allow us to find peace for the lives we have lead, the future of the lives to come. I hope to help my clients find peace within our sessions and tools to allow the self-healing to continue once we are finished.

Always studding, ready and willing to learn new skills to aid and add to my trade, I take pride knowing that when you are in my space and energy I am there for you warts and all.

As a mother of two strong-willed, thunderous, big beautiful hearted boys (12 and 9), I am giving what I believe to be the right foundations to be compassionate, wise, caring loving men.

I ask you, what have you done for yourself that has made you feel amazing? If you can't answer that, I encourage you to see you the way your higher self sees you. It starts from within then the love and vibration can cascade out and flow to others. You are the love you deserve.

Blessings to you Soul Warrior

www.lunahealing.com.au/
Facebook: Luna-Healing-106779024837940 & groups/121605308543354

Kubarli Dreaming

Heidi Mippy

She comes to me as I close my eyes. Her wailing dances to the rhythm of tapping sticks. Face painted like a spirit. Slowly she begins to move; palms open, knees bent, she's close to the ground, moving so peacefully, her eyes staring back at me, her aura lighting up the dark place. She sings to me 'warlu, warluuuu'. Her feet beat the ground in time, sand flicks up in a dusty cloud, tears roll down her cheeks. She stands still. Her spirit lifts to the sky to rest. She is home.
Annali Mippy-Smith (Daughter -15 years of age)

I am standing on country. The soles of my bare feet are planted on the granite rocks that protect and cleanse the sacredness of the water that surrounds me. I begin to cry, the tears feel cool as they slowly run down my warm face, the wind kissing them as it works its way through the big marri trees. The tears are heavier now and I feel a sense of pain. A pain that only a mother can feel when she loses her child. As I sit with this feeling, I speak to the spirits that are around me, I speak to country and I am open to what they want me to see. Before my eyes, I see the most beautiful dark-skinned women from this country, from many moons ago. Their dark flawless skin is covered in red ochre. It covers their bare chests, roughly painted onto their breasts and across their stomach. The women are conducting a ceremony in the water. They are washing their daughters part naked bodies in the cool, fresh water. As the ochre runs off their bodies, tears fall and their wailing can be heard and felt as a vibration through the river, in the air, and across the land. I look up now towards the outcrops overlooking the river. Here I can see the men, they are from the rivers further south. They are waiting for the women to do their business. They stand on the hill alone, but they will leave with their new wives, whose blood now flows through to the very rivers that run through the men's homelands. The noise of the white-tailed cockatoo breaks my vision and shows me the totem of the children who will be born from this ceremony. I feel happy now. Content. But my responsibility for this starts here. With this vision and awareness, I am now obliged to share and protect the space. Honour this story.

I am Aboriginal. I am Indigenous. I am First Nations. I am all those labels that you may know or have come to understand but I identify according to the tribes to which I belong. I am a Thiin-Mah Warrianygka and Noongar woman. This means I have an ancestral connection to the Upper Gascoyne and South West regions of Western Australia. My old people have walked this country, cared for, and sustained it for tens of thousands of years. My story began in Carnarvon where the saltwater meets the freshwater. My soul most comes to life when I am close to these waters. When I am far away from the saltwater I crave it so badly that I can taste the salt on my lips and my tongue. This is one way that country talks to me, and sings me where she wants me to go. I always listen because she knows best. If I don't listen, she finds a way to make me pay attention!

Fresh water rivers in secluded parts of the bush are where I find myself most connected to my soul, where my heart sings the most beautiful tune and where the layers of the everyday world instantly strip away, piece by piece to reveal me, the authentic me, the me I like to connect with every day, the me I like to be. There is something about water that is nurturing and healing but also strangely sensual. It is where my feminine energy is highly aroused. Some of the most beautiful intimate moments I have had, have been in and around water. Normally I wouldn't share those things but given this space, I choose to sit in that power and honour these experiences as they have honoured me. Some might refer to this talk as women's business but I disagree because there are magical moments between men and women that are sacred, but are also meant to be talked about between both genders. I call this everyone's business although this doesn't mean I would go telling the world all the details. Instead, I mean this to be that men and women should be encouraged to talk with each other about these experiences safely and healthily, knowing and understanding each other's souls and bodies, and how to respectfully bring pleasure to self and each other. I long for the day when my People do this more freely, breaking down the barriers of modern interpretations of men's and women's business and smashing through intergenerational trauma so that we can re-establish the healthy, unconditional love for self and others we have known since time first existed.

When I first saw the title of this book 'Rising Matriarch', I was immediately drawn to the project. Matriarch has such a deep meaning to me that goes well beyond any dictionary definition or label. By the way, I hate labels. A single word never does justice. When I hear the word matriarch I feel the spirits of my old people standing beside me. I connect with culture and spirit, with wisdom and power, I feel safe, loved, and guided. I feel responsibility and obligation. I see and taste the water; the giver of life and I see a oneness that brings this all together. I see and feel a woman standing in her power. It might have been that the reason I was drawn to this project was that I had just been through a horrific experience, where my power and my life were almost taken from me, by the hands of the father of my two eldest children. It might have been because the past year I had been silenced in a relationship with a man who I am in love with, but due to his trauma, was restricting what I could communicate, when and how. I just needed to bring myself back into a space where I felt I was in control of my life, my feelings and to be free to be me. Either way, I was determined to be part of it and nothing can stop a determined blak woman!

I am a mother of three beautiful girls. I am fierce but I am gentle. I am proud but I am humble. I am loving and I am powerful. I am the backbone of my family. I don't like the label of a single mother – to me it implies many stereotypes that I do not feel comfortable with and I have had labels and stereotypes thrown at me my entire life. So I am not a single mother, I am a mother who has raised all her children, for the majority of their lives, on her own. I am a warrior. I am a matriarch but I find myself asking if I am a rising matriarch and if so, what am I rising from? When did I come into my power? Have I come into my power? These are questions I have sat with many times.

I believe that being in our power changes and evolves like the wind and the tides. I became who I am not entirely by choice but absolutely with a shitload of determination. I am who I am because of my lived experiences and that which has been handed down to me through the lived experiences of my ancestors. And I continue to grow with the lived experiences of my children. I own my power, it belongs to me, but it is not always within my control. There are times I am weak and I am vulnerable. There are times I have been down and defeated. There are times I have second-guessed and not felt my worth. My story in this space isn't about my trauma and rising from the ashes. It is about the intergenerational trauma, the resilience, and the wisdom that has shaped me through life and has made me who I am.

My contribution to this book was shown to me, as part of my obligation to those who have journeyed before me, those who are present in my world today, and those who will be here in the future, long after I am gone. It is a cultural obligation that matriarchs from my People carry, being a mother or not. This is women's business, it is men's business and it is everyone's business. It is the balance of all these things, the trilogy of life. My power is not without the influences of men. Without balance, the trilogy of life and our existence is lost and damaged, and this is felt and seen in our community in the form of hurt and trauma. I feel I am able and obligated to restore this balance in several ways, one being through sharing my story and allowing my voice to be heard.

For a long time, I often felt I had been silenced. Physically, spiritually and sexually. I believe intergenerational trauma has played a massive part, but of course, it has only recently been recognised and still doesn't receive the attention it should. Let me unpack this a little so you might understand where I am coming from.

I belong to the most beautiful ancient culture in this world yet in my time, women have too often been silenced. Destructive and self-destructive behaviours surrounded my childhood and extended through to my adulthood. Growing up was a bitch! There was no clear rite of passage, just constant navigation through a cruel and confusing world. As a young person, I saw girls looking for sex, when in fact what they were looking for was self-worth and love that they were unable to find at home or within. As a young woman, I was shown that it was not ok to assert myself, be the boss of my house or hold down a career. Women in my community, have been treated like sex objects by men (that is someone to have sex with), and the gift of a child is considered greater than love. You should count yourself lucky if you become a baby Mumma! Women in my community have treated other women equally as poorly as men. Jealously, violence, lateral violence. These destructive behaviours are a reflection of intergenerational trauma; hurt people hurting people. This has been my life. You see this play out now in the form of joint Facebook accounts, where there is one identity and you don't even know who is posting, or which person in the relationship likes pineapple on their pizza but you know one of them does! One thing you can be sure of, is they don't trust each other to have separate accounts, their own friends, and their own identity and relationships. If you were to ask, they would tell you that it's easier to have the one account, and they are both happy to be sharing, but who are they kidding?

For me, I hate the thought of my voice and rights being taken away from me. I have been the target of countless attempts at casual sex by men, that were so loaded with aggression, I began to fear men! Sex was never a challenge for me, the challenge I set for myself was to not engage in these destructive behaviours, hold my power and my worth. Don't get me wrong, I haven't got this right all the time. There have been times I have faltered and learned some lessons. But overall, I have always understood that during sex the exchange of both high and low vibrational energy was present, and I was very aware of its impact on me. It didn't interest me to experience endless moments of these exchanges of energy, nor to be in competition with anyone else.

As a result of my choices, many men think I am stuck up and love myself.

They assume I think I'm too good for them and above them because I refuse to have sex with them. Then I dared to become educated, have a career and sit in this weird healing space, which is conveniently misunderstood but is and always will be, part of our ancient ways.

It's a fuck of a place to be. Damned if you do, damned if you don't. But all I have ever wanted was to connect with someone culturally, spiritually, and energetically; and if it were the right circumstances then sex would follow, and so would some deep connections that would allow growth. There was always a spiritual element to sex and relationships that I yearned for, and as I have gotten older, I no longer sacrifice that desire. I want young girls to know they don't have to sacrifice themselves too.

As a mother of three girls, I don't want them to grow up with the inherent jealousy, abuse, and bullying that I have experienced, and which is far too common. I never dared to shine my light, constantly dimming it down in fear of someone having a go at me. These days I just don't give a fuck. I do me. I don't try to outshine others but I will not hesitate to shine my light and hold my own space and hold space for others. I know who I am and who I am not. For this reason, it is hard to find a man, particularly a Noongar man who respects me and isn't intimidated by me. But why should I settle for anything less? Why is self-love so difficult and hate so easy? Why are joint Facebook accounts so common? I don't want my girls used and abused and disrespected by anyone. I don't want them to use and abuse themselves. So I devote my time to holding space for others to connect with themselves and shift through the trauma that is causing them to hurt themselves and hurt others. I hold space for others to learn to love themselves and connect with self and spirit.

Culture is intervention, and culture and country help us to heal. I know that most of you reading this book will resonate with the healing power of country; sitting under a majestic ancient tree, watching and listening to the birds fly over, feeling the wind on your face, or planting your feet into the sand. You wouldn't have been drawn to this book if you didn't understand this.

In our contemporary culture, we have this thing called shame that far too often gets in the way of young people being the best they can be. Shame holds our young ones back because it inhibits them from growing and shining their light. We hide behind shame instead of challenging ourselves and daring to be. Society then sets expectations far too low for our young people and today's culture of systemic disadvantage, racism, and intergenerational trauma adds far too many layers of complexity for our young people who are just trying to 'be.' Every day is a fight for me, to ensure my children have access to their best life. I will fight until the day I die, just like my old people did.

In my younger years, I was one of those people who was self-conscious and shy. Most people today would call bullshit on that because that isn't what they see and maybe that isn't what they saw back then, but that is exactly who I was. I never liked the attention of people and remember being bullied and teased more than I ever felt loved and supported. As a mother, I don't want my kids to ever feel that and I have always fought to give them the safest home, the best opportunities, lots of love, and encouraged them to shine. I have not got this right every time. I have made choices that made my life harder so I could give my girls the best, but I have no regrets. Everything has happened just as it was meant to. Life isn't meant to be easy, it is meant to be understood, and in understanding comes knowing; most importantly knowing self.

My Nan was a staunch woman born in 1928 and bore the brunt of Australia's darkest history. Legislative acts that denied her and her family the rights to practice culture, to be free, to be respected, to be themselves. She always taught me that if I wanted something I had to work hard for it, to not expect handouts, and to get a good education because a good education is how you successfully walk in two worlds. I took her advice because I felt her love and saw her wisdom. She was the matriarch of our family and I honour her story through my own. Today, I am grateful to have had her guidance because, without the education, experience, and qualifications that I have, I would not have been able to raise my kids free from welfare and dependency. I would not have been able to overcome barriers and stereotypes continually imposed upon my people. I would not have had the freedom or fight within, to work hard for myself and my people. This is the impact of a matriarch. She is powerful, she is amazing, she does not need to be present in this world to shift mountains.

Today I am forty-one years old. I have spent a lot of time over the past years, coming to know and love myself. I have worked through identified trauma and become comfortable with a raised consciousness and awareness. I no longer deny my spirituality and connection to spirit, I embrace it. Up until now, I have never wanted to be married. This isn't to say that I have never been in love because I have, but I have considered marriage a space where I would become one and lose my independence, identity, and name! I have been fiercely independent because I have seen too many abusive and controlling relationships where both women and men are lost. As a woman who has built her career, raised her children and relied on nobody else, it's a scary thought to be dependent on another and risk everything that you have worked so hard for, including your children. I have suffered losses because I have made choices to remove myself from relationships that were not serving a purpose for me and my children. I have lost houses, money, I have lost my dignity. I have put myself in painful hardships to protect myself and my children and to keep on a path moving forward. And in the darkest of hours, the depths of despair, I have had the voice of my old people guiding me, showing me that there is a greater purpose and to keep moving, and because of that I have.

One of these voices is my Pop. I could write an entire book about this man; I love him deeply. I was ten years old when he passed but I can feel his presence today, just like he is still here. I value men. I know that men have a critical role to play in our lives, our culture, and our society. My Pop often appears to growl me, at times when I am being too independent, or being taken advantage of. He calls me his Noongar Princess, which makes me laugh because I am far from a princess and his parting words are always 'keep doing what makes your heart sing'. My Nan and Pop are like yin and yang. One talks to me from a space of sense and responsibility and the other talks from the heart, spirit, and culture. This has given me balance and I have valued the learnings they have gifted me both in their living years and spirit. My Pop has helped me to hold on to the faith that the right man will enter my world at the right time. He will be a beautiful, loving man with a gentle soul but a strong will to be able to understand and appreciate my fierce independence and put up with me! He will not want to control my life or ask for a joint Facebook account, instead, he will add value to it, his strengths overcoming my weaknesses, my strengths overcoming his weaknesses. His gentleness breaking down the walls I have built. His soul will dance with mine well before we meet and when we make love our souls will unite on the deepest levels and deepen both our understanding of self, each other, and life. He will love and honour his Matriarchs and as a result, he will love and honour me and my children. And this will close the circle in my life. Freeing me from independence and survival mode. The balance sending ripples far and wide into our community.

I am part of a nation of sleeping giants and I believe we, as a People are rising and coming into our power; reinstating the power and position of women. This is Kubarli (Grandmother) Dreaming.

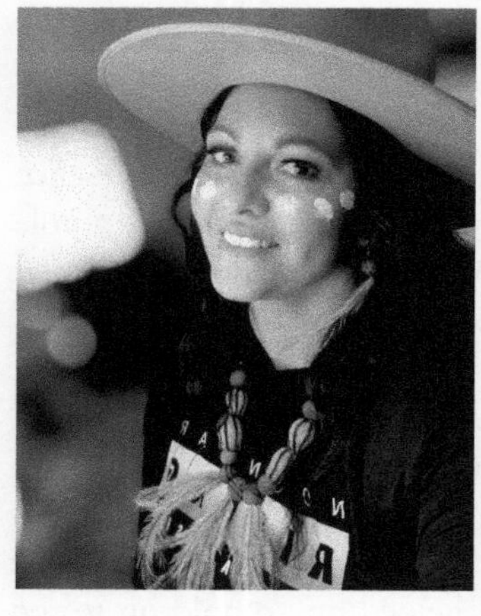

Heidi Mippy

Well this is certainly a big honour for me to be in this space, surrounded by so many amazing women. I want to start by paying my respects to the First Nations people from the lands on which this book has journeyed to. I want to acknowledge the continued power and beauty that the ancient people bring to each and every one of our lives and experiences. I give love and gratitude to my old people, both men and women who have walked this land before me but wish to acknowledge the strength of the matriarchs who have been the key to holding our culture alive for tens of thousands of years. My name is Heidi Mippy and I am proud Noongar, Thiin-Mah Warriangyka warrior. I am a mother. I have three beautiful, amazing, unique, powerful, resilient, warriors of my own. The matriarchs of our family live on and through each of us. We stand on the shoulders of giants and we walk humbly but proudly in our culture, our place and identity as women. I am a healer. I create, I inspire, I lead, I hold space for others as I share my gifts and help bring balance and perspective to this world. I have done this as a professional in the many roles that I have held but I also do this as a person, through my business, as a consultant and in my personal time and spaces, but especially out on country where I know the power of healing is seen, felt, and heard more easily than amongst the hustle and bustle of everyday life.

Instagram: @matriarchdreaming
Facebook: matriarchdreaming
LinkedIn: heidi-mippy

The Wild Within

K P Weaver

Darkness is all I saw, even though my eyes were wide open. The shock of the loss of the 'perfect' life I worked hard to maintain shook me to my core, and I was caught in the grip of PTSD.

Day by day was the only way to move through each empty moment. I never knew what it felt to feel nothing before and I stayed there too long. A year was too long to be in this cocoon so eventually universal intervention was bound to happen, and it did in the wake-up call of a gruelling double miscarriage. I cried buckets of tears for the babies I loved and lost and also for the lost year beforehand.

So, what was I to do? Let the past year and all its darkness define the rest of my life and become a bitter victim of circumstance? Hell no!

I did the opposite and took all the wisdom I accumulated from a year-long journey inward. I was more connected to myself; inhibitions were nowhere to be found and I was passionate and courageous with what I was planning. After being in a cocoon for a year, I was ready to live again. I set some big intentions!

I decided that if I was going to have any more children I wanted to get married. Having a different name than my children didn't float my boat anymore. This was a huge change for me as I NEVER wanted to let go of my maiden name of Weaver. I loved it so much I always said I would never get married, but it was time. This shift altered something in me and I was ready to embrace another identity for a while. That's what I believe happens when we get married and take on another name, our identity is altered and it either serves us or it doesn't. For me, for now, it served me. I remember going to visit a numerologist in 2009 and she did a chart on my married name and one on my maiden name. I knew the difference as I wore both hats daily.

When I lost the twins, all I remember was two long weeks trying to save one, but alas, my prayers were not enough and I lost them both.

I couldn't bear the emptiness in my womb, I prayed for a miracle, and I got it! I know now that I was manifesting the gift that was to come. I was determined to pass the spiritual test, the test I speak about later when I wrote my first novel The Visitor.

I was pregnant within a month! To this day I do not remember doing the deed needed to make it happen because, to be honest, it was the last thing on my mind after the trauma I had endured over the two weeks I was losing my twins. But it happened; she is my rainbow child and I was not going to question it. I remember going very slow for 3 months. I found out very early that I was pregnant and I did life gently until I reached the milestone. Though it was not easy, as I had a wedding to organise in a few short months.

Then life had another major event for us to embrace. The day I was picking up our wedding rings from the jewellers, I got a call from our emigration company saying that our Australian visas had been processed. It was amazing. Even though I was expecting, had just finished building a new house and was about to get married, I never waivered from the Knowing that we were to move to Australia.

It was tough to leave. I am very close to my sister and with another grandchild so close to being born my mum and dad were of course very conflicted in thier emotions. On one hand they wanted a better life for me, and on the other, they didn't want to lose me and my family.

I was 35 weeks pregnant the day I got on the plane, destination down under. I had to get a special letter from the hospital to say that I could fly. I waddled up and down the plane every hour of the 20-hour flight. When we arrived on the first day of spring 2008 we knew no one. We had two nights booked in a motel on the Great Eastern Highway and a lot to organise so that we could get settled in before my baby was to arrive.

Giving birth in Australia was such a beautiful experience compared to delivering my boys in Ireland. With both boys, I went ten days over and so had to be induced. It was a very clinical experience with a drip and not the natural experience I had in Australia with only my waters being broke, before giving birth naturally. I have a very strong sack, one that never wanted to let me have the feeling of waters being broken. One of my daughters was born in her sack; with my last child, my waters broke on a Sunday morning. It was my sixth child and yet I didn't know what had just happened.

I adored being a mum at home with my kids, but in 2010 the call came to write. It was loud and clear and I couldn't ignore it. I had just had my fourth child, and while watching The View, I had an epiphany when Whoopi Goldberg shared some resonating words with a celebrity TV couple. The wild within me was calling. I was soon to realise the power of the written word.

I told my husband, 'for the next 30 days you do not have a wife! I'm going to write a novel during NanoWrimo' (National novel writing month that happens every November). And so being the best mum I could be whilst staying dedicated to writing 1667 words a day for 30 days, I wrote a novel with my story woven through it. I don't know where it came from, or how the story flowed and the characters developed. I wasn't a novelist, but I didn't block myself by overthinking, I was committed to my first draft and what it would be. I let it organically take shape every day for 30 days and I got a certificate when I uploaded all 51000 words on November 30, 2010.

Little did I know then that the journey was just beginning. Every book takes you on a journey, one with huge potential if you allow it. I went through a self-publishing journey with a publisher in the US. It was all about money and not very much about my book. I was a novice, and I didn't have a clue what I was to be doing. I was resentful towards them, when I looked at my newly published book and thought, *Wow that was not worth it!* Then one day something clicked in me that shifted my perspective altogether. I had learned a lot about the process of publishing and in taking some inspiration from the quote at the very start of my book, *From every negative situation is the potential for a positive outcome*, I chose to research the print and distribution channel that my publisher used, only to discover that they had opened an office in Melbourne that very month. I made a promise to myself that if I was accepted as a publisher with them then I would answer the call to help stories be shared in the world and help others have a positive publishing experience alongside writing and publishing my own stories. **I reclaimed my power in that moment.**

The fire within was fuelled with so much passion for what I was doing. People were coming to me and I would help them get published, but I also did something more, I really cared. A writing and publishing journey is an evolutionary process and always comes with hurdles to overcome so that advancement will occur. Before every breakthrough there is always a struggle.

I became more and more confident as I surged forward in this high vibrational energy, all the time having babies along the way. I have six children in total and that is where I stop. Something happens to my body, heart and mind every time I have a child. The loving intention and glow I have around the birth of a child is the most divine and pure energy and I have come to love to write in this energy. I realised that love was the most powerful energy of all and that when I put loving intention into something it supercharged it and I got results in record times. So I started setting huge intentions and fuelled them with loving energy. I would scatter many intention seeds and some would take hold, some wouldn't and that was ok.

To date, I have written and published 40 of my own books in many genres including children's non-fiction, fiction and journals. I'm called a multi-genre author, which is wonderful, but my passion for story is driven by the impact words have on people when they need to read them. And that mission has seen me go on the most epic life adventure and I pinch myself every day.

I am not going to say it has all been rosy but I make a conscious decision every day to get out on the right side of the bed, and delve into life positively. It's a choice that takes energy, and every day I reap the rewards from it. It works for me a high majority of the time but as I said it doesn't come easy, I have had to fight for this choice. Not everyone around me wants to live in the bright shiny light I produce. I live fiercely through the power of the written word. I know what happens when words connect and I fuel my energy into that channel every day because my mission, my calling, is to help get stories told. When a story connects to someone who needs to read it, it shifts something in them and that shift has a ripple effect in their life and the lives of countless others around them.

From the exterior I have had HUGE success, and by my own definition, which is to prioritise my happiness, do what I love and be a great mum who is present as much as possible, I reckon that I am successful in many ways. But what many people don't know is that the wild woman within me was fuelled by a stubbornness that arose from a really tough relationship with my husband.

One of the things I have come to realise in life is that you can't make someone else happy unless they choose that they want to be happy. Just because I prioritise happiness doesn't mean that someone else does. Once I freed myself from that thought and the expectation of myself to spend my precious time on someone who didn't deserve it, and start to focus on the things that I could have a positive impact on (hello my children and business), then things began to shift for the better.

My relationship is something I have silently struggled with for years, because I always try to see the good in people, I always try to find the positive in the negative and I never want to change that trait about me.

In the past thirteen years (since moving to Australia), my main struggle has been in my relationship. I have been through many cycles, and many horrible situations, one where I had to flee my house with my kids in the middle of the night. And yet, I absolutely still value the importance of having dad around, and so I did everything I could to keep our home together and keep myself sane by focusing on building my businesses and being a mum.

There were a few years when I was not in my power. Looking back now I can't believe some of it, but I know my intentions were always laser-focused on doing the right thing for all of us. Standing here today I know I have done my best, because I honoured the Wild call from within and trust every decision that I have made. Even though I have experienced some very dark moments, I never shy away from the deep core growth that shines through them. I don't do the victim well and I also don't do being quiet well, and so I say to any woman who feels that they have no power: *Please find that one thing that you do have power over, something that fits you well. Find something that you enjoy doing and find a way to do it, it will keep you alive inside. Fight for it, it is worth fighting for. It is your way out!*

For other people looking in on someone else's life, please know that everything looks and feels so different when you are inside the box. Try not to judge someone you love, who you see in the box. Give them a smile, a safe place where they can show up and share without you taking action. That will help them build up the strength they need to grow and take positive action. Personally I am not a person who enjoys conflict. I love to have a high vibe, and peaceful equilibrium, but I have come to realise the importance of some healthy conflict in initiating positive change, especially in a relationship.

And if you meet a brick wall and criticism every time you have a win or success, go somewhere else to celebrate. That is actively choosing to take positive action in your life because you can choose who you happy dance with.

I have though, grown and trust my *Knowing* so much, that no amount of criticism can penetrate it. I've done the hard work. I've honoured my divine goddess inside and answered the call to live my purpose, and because of this I now listen to the narrative I tell myself. I know what I want out of life and I go for it with all my heart, but not just for me. I do it for my children, and for everyone I inspire to find themselves and shine through that. And although it is not *all* for me, I also do it for me because if I keep my cup full I will continue to give my best to the world.

I encourage everyone reading this, no matter what your external circumstances are, to please honour the wild within. It is here to serve you and will gift you all the strength you need to help you reach your highest purpose.

And then by living in my divine, wild go-getting goddess, loving my children, and living my best-self, something truly amazing happened. My partner awoke and started to see life from a different place. And all of a sudden everything is ok again.

Don't compromise on your purpose or on your core values. Be steadfast, go after what it is that you want, stand in that divine power with love and be true to you! Embrace the wild within because she has your back.

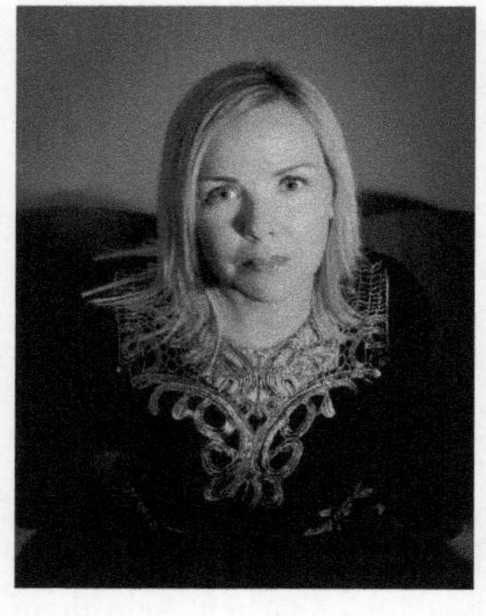

K P Weaver

Hello hello, I wear two hats. One as K P Weaver and one as Karen Mc Dermott. The reason for that is because I am both an author and a publisher and I need to keep a clear boundary between them, both in my mind and in my branding. Karen Mc Dermott, the publisher is way more confident but K P Weaver is catching up!

I have been writing since 2010 when I penned my first novel The Visitor in 30 days during the annual challenge NanoWrimo. I caught the writing bug in that moment and could happily sit and write all day every day, in fact, my end goal is to have a house on a hill with a bay window, gorgeous view and an open-door policy for my grown-up kids to come and go as they please. I suspect this might be based in Ireland, but it might just as well be Australia too.

I have been a publisher since 2012 when I founded Serenity Press first as a hybrid press and then as a traditional press in 2016. I went on to found MMH Press in 2016 and KMD books in 2019. My publishing academy was founded to support authors in a group environment and I love showing up in this group and seeing all of the goodness that happens in there.

As proud mum of 6 I am blessed to have buckets loads of love to go around. My children are my world and I never take for granted that I am blessed to do what I do alongside being a hands-on mum. They grow up way to fast!

I absolutely believe in the magic of life and I choose a positive lifestyle every day. My Life Magic with K P Weaver group is a Facebook group where we focus on the positives, the universal laws and releasing any blocks to greatness and you are invited to join too.

www.karenweaverauthor.com
www.kpweaver.com
www.serenitypress.org
www.mmhpress.com
www.kmdbooks.com
www.everythingpublishingacademy.com

Unapologetically You…

Wild, Wise & Free

Kathryn Ottobrino

My entire life, I feel like I have been put in a BOX; a small restrictive box that makes me want to scream from the top of my lungs. AND my chest feels so heavy when I have found myself back in this place at different times on my life journey, and through different experiences it seems to feel even more restrictive …

Told to follow rules, told to keep my voice down, told to do things this way, told to follow what is deemed societal acceptable, told I am making bad choices, told I need to fix myself, told to not to speak my truth or I may upset someone, even told to get married, told to buy a house and have kids … told to stop living life on my terms. Arghhhhhhh even writing that brings back so many hard, challenging, extremely lonely, PAINFUL and confusing times in my life.

I mean who came up with these boxes anyway … and what right do they have to tell anyone how they should be living their life. Yes that's right, the human experience I am having right now as I write this chapter … didn't we arrive here as sovereign beings? Our souls decided to come down and have a human experience …

So from a very young age, I feel I subconsciously decided to create my own BOX and follow my own rules. I was always the one causing some sort of rebellious trouble, the one that refused to be told what to do, the one that everyone knew had a big mouth. But all that really was, in hindsight, was me sharing my own individual truth and not caring what anyone thought …

Growing up though I knew I was different, I knew that I had such deep innate soul wisdom that was bursting to come out of me and share it with the world. I also had such a strong intuition and could read people's energies and feel their emotions within a few minutes of meeting them. But for so long I suppressed this, as I was trying hard to fight my way out of the box I was told to stay in, I now fully accept that one of my superpowers is my intuition and use it very wisely in my life and to my advantage.

As I grew older and more aware, this led me to consciously choosing my own box every single day, yes that's right, the rules of my soul. I got so tired of being told 'I WAS TOO MUCH' and 'TO FOLLOW THE RULES' AND feeling like there was something wrong with me day in and day out, which then led me to making decisions based on what I 'should be doing in life.'

So, enough was enough and I made a sacred commitment to only listen to my own inner guidance and always be LED BY SOUL … my own soul and no-one else's … to embrace me. Lets be honest, we all have our own unique inner soul and guidance that no-one can and will ever properly understand the intracacy of your soul.

However this wasn't alway the case and I spent many days wishing I could hide and mask parts of myself; trying to understand what the hell was wrong with me.

These words haunted me most days for years.

Tame it down Kathryn.

Censor yourself..

You are too much Kathryn.

In a nutshell, what that means is "DON'T BE YOURSELF KATHRYN"

This led to the start of what I now know was my journey with anxiety and depression; the constant wondering 'why am I so different' and 'how can I be normal?' A journey that I have had to live with my entire adult life and still continue to manage this every day.

I was always in reactive mode trying to justify myself and explain why I was doing what I was doing. Explaining why I was making certain decisions that only my soul knew was the right one.

Like when she (my soul) told me to move to Tokyo at seventeen, leave one of the most isolated cities in the world where i grew up, to spread my wings and take a job with a local newspaper. My parents were not impressed let me tell you!. Holy shit that sounded bat shit crazy to most people, yes get on a plane and move to a foreign country on the other side of the world where people barely spoke English. But I knew I had to do this, and I knew it was part of the first of many spiritual awakenings for me. This adventure for me was the start of the beginning of living life following the soul nudges and what an eye opening experience it was.

Or when she told me to move to London at twenty-two and travel and explore Europe with just a backpack and no end date. This led me to continue living in London for nearly five years and create a new life for myself there.

Or when she told me to use every last penny I had, to the point where rent was not going to be paid that week, so that I could fly to another state and do a self-development course, a course which changed my life forever and skyrocketed me into my soul's purpose. doing what I believe I was sent here to do, spread light and SHARE MY SOUL'S WISDOM.

Or when she told me to pack up all my belongings in 2016 while I was living in Melbourne, become totally location free, wander around life like a gypsy; no home, no stability just going with the flow. Now that's where I really learnt the art of total trust and surrender. More on that topic below.

Or when she guided me to fall in love with a man from another country, while he was visiting my then current city Sydney. Then continued to explore a long distant relationship with him while knowing it would probably never be possible for us to be together long-term, but still following the nudges.

Or when she guided me to move to Bali and live a life of complete freedom, to claim everything I wanted and let go of everything I had, to start again. A story I know so well.

And the list goes on. These are just some of the many life altering and absolutely mind-blowing experiences that life has presented me with because I threw out the rule books and created my own guide. The guide that allows me to be wild, wise and free, in all my mess.

However, while I talk so courageously and loosely about these fun, soul-led experiences, let me now talk about what I have personally had to overcome to keep this sacred commitment to my soul, and the many challenges and the constant adversity that I am still faced with in my present life.

Yes here is the reality of being me and choosing to live a life led by soul, a life where no-one has any influence over me but me. A life that I get to choose every single day, not one that chooses me.

Firstly let's talk about the dreaded F word, FEAR.

Let me start by asking you this question. Do you think Fear will just suddenly go away one day? Like puff, just be gone and never come back?

Good because the short answer is no and I am going to talk about how to navigate your way through facing fear so that you can, and always will, be led by your soul …

But first and foremost let's talk about that F word that so many people dread and try to avoid at all costs throughout their life.

For so many years I did this exact thing and tried to avoid any situations that would present me with any fear. I was so scared of losing control that I played it safe. But the thing is, I was so unfulfilled and felt like my soul was dying inside.

Once I realised that fear was here to stay until the day I left my physical body, I decided to explore deeper and start learning ways to live with it and cultivate a relationship with it that served me and my big dreams, desires and goals.

It wasn't an overnight thing and still to this day I experience fear, but I face and embrace it differently, and I hope after reading this you will too … why? Because fear will prevent you from living a life that is led by your soul and will try to control your every move if you let it.

And fear gets louder and bigger the more you start taking big leaps of faith and moving towards your soul's desires. It thinks it is keeping you safe but it may be controlling your life so much that you won't be able to live a fulfilled happy life the way you imagined.

I am going to talk more about this later in the chapter but I want you let this statement land, "Let fear in, see it, feel it , be with it and simply love it."

Whatever you do, don't let fear take the driver's seat, or be in charge of the directions, just simply let it be there; just by your side, be kind to it, but be assertive with it because your soul is in charge here.

Everytime I have fear come up I get really honest with what the truth is. I ask myself, 'is this the truth?' or, "Is this here to show me the way, to show me what's possible?'

And I choose to release the fear and choose trust and surrender.

Yes, now let's talk all about trust and surrender. For so many years I lived in such a state of fear and control. It wasn't until I really started listening to my own soul's guidance did I really have to lean into what this looked like. People would say 'just trust the path,' and it would infuriate me so much as I wanted to know exactly what was going to happen in every moment.

The more I started to build a healthy relationship with fear, the more I started to explore what trust and surrender looked like for me and how to start to build a rock-solid relationship with it.

I used to get to levels of trust and surrender, only to realise I was still in my logical mind and there were parts of me that were trying to control outcomes.

Things would show up for me in my outside reality to show me I wasn't really in a surrender state. Things I didn't necessary like as the universe was trying to give me signs to let go even more. The more you try to micro-manage the universe, the more you will be met with resistance.

When you have your own back, trust and surrender, and know that you are safe and supported at all times, expect all kinds of magic moments to walk through your door.

But leaning into the deepest levels of trust and surrender requires you to embody a feeling that looks a bit like, 'attached to nothing but connected to everything.' It is a feeling and a state of vibration that washes over you; a sense of calmness that I can't even put into words.

Every time I knew I was being called forward and asked to lean more into this state and vibration, I would immerse myself in nature and ground back into my body; dance has also been a really a really supportive tool for me to step into this. We cannot get to this state from being in our mind, we have to embody it within our body.

I know how scary it is to live in uncertainty, trust me I have been beside myself many times, scared shitless things would fall apart and not work out the way I imagined, but every time they worked out bigger and better than ever. There are those magic moments again.

Are you holding on too tight and blocking what magic moments want to show up for you? At some point there comes a time when you have to surrender and let go of trying to micro-manage and control every single outcome and life experience.

It may be the hardest thing you'll ever have to lean into, but it is one of the most expansive things you can do for yourself. In each and every moment be open to miracles and magic moments that want to show up for you.

Surrender into being unapologetically you
Surrender into being wild, wise and free

I want to share some other words of wisdom and nuggets that I have had to learn over the many years of making a commitment to follow my soul's compass and being unapologeticly me.

It comes with doing things that are really uncomfortable at times.
It comes with having extremely strong boundaries.
It comes with going all in on this vision of freedom and doing what it takes.
It comes with asking for support and having a tribe of people by my side.
It comes with backing myself all day, everyday.
It comes with adversity and deep challenges.
It comes with breaking the rules of society.
It comes with not always having financial stability.
It comes with investing in myself time & time again.
It comes with having daily practices that are non-negotiable.
It comes with bloody hard yards at times.

It comes with being of service to humanity even when I am in my own shit because that is my SOUL'S purpose.

So let's go back to where I started this chapter..

My entire life I feel like I have been put in a box ...

Some days …
Some days I wish I wasn't so open.
Some days I wish I wasn't so vulnerable.
Some days I wish I wasn't so real & raw with what I share with the world.
Some days I wish I wasn't so powerful.
Some days I wish I wasn't me.
Some days I wish I didn't care what people think.
Some days I wish my 'not good enough story' didn't surface.
Some days I wish I wasn't so confident & comfortable in who I am.
Some days I wonder why I am even here feeling so much pain.
Some days I am so lonely I could hide forever.
Some days I feel so broken and lost.

But most days I feel so alive and free and the fear takes a hike.
And I take huge leaps of faith to keep leaning into new wedges of me.
I feel free just being me, and all of me.
No one else but me, the sovereign soul I came here to be, flaws and all, with courage only some will understand.
No masks.
No hiding.
No censuring.
No pretending.
Sharing the real me.
The too much side of me.
The good ,the bad ,the RAW.
The uncomfortable.
The softer side.
The deepest parts of my soul.

She is wild, wise & free
She is strong but soft
She is judged but secure
She is empowered but vulnerable
She is brave but scared
She is shining her light, but faces darkness
She is grounded but fierce
She is open but closed
She is spiritual but sass
She is intuitive but Intelligent
She is flow but force

She is confident but calm
She is desirable & deserving
She is powerful & potent
She is inspiring & igniting
She is surrendered but safe
She is multi-dimensional but integrated
She is too much but truthful
She is raw but real
She is abundant & aligned
She is intentional but unpredictable
She is polarised but perfect
She is hurt but hopeful
She is trusting when she feels safe
She is awakened but aware
She is seen … she is supported

What would it take for you to be all of you?

For you to love and accept all parts and not care what anyone thinks. To lean into the edges and show up as the imperfect soul that you came here to be.

To be wild, wise and free

To be imperfect

Inner Freedom lives right here.

To face the shadow parts of yourself and to then bring them to the light to shine even brighter. It's too much for some I get it, It can shine a light on where they may be hiding parts of themselves behind closed doors, and disowning parts because it's deemed to be 'unacceptable' (that story can take a hike I say).

Where they are too scared and extremely uncomfortable to be ALL OF THEM … But you get to show them how it is done, to be unapologetically you.

To speak your truth with love, integrity,ease and grace and not be scared that you will be judged or shamed.

Inner Freedom lives right here.

I am going to leave you with the the lyrics of 'I am me.' It always hits me so deep & hard every time I listen to it, and I want you to know that you can be unapologetically you, WILD,WISE AND FREE … owning all parts of you.

I am me
I am brave, I am bruised
I am who I'm meant to be, this is me
Look out 'cause here I come
And I'm marching on to the beat I drum

I'm not scared to be seen
I make no apologies, this is me
I see you
I feel you
I was you

With love Kat x

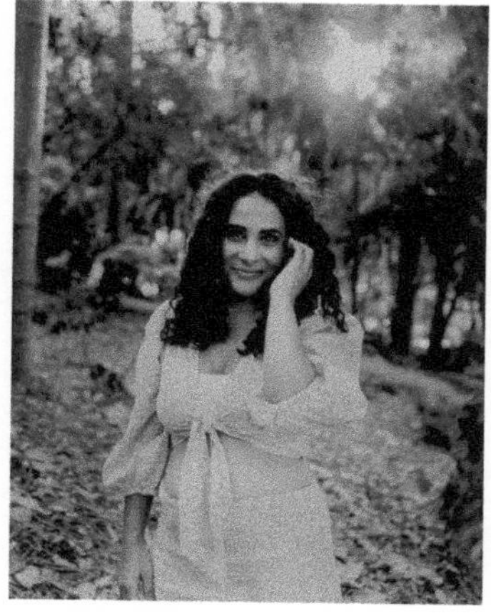

Kathryn Ottobrino

Hi I'm Kathryn Ottobrino, a Spiritual Business Mentor, Soul Coach, Intuitive Healer, Speaker, Neuro-Linguistic Programming (NLP) / Emotional Freedom Technique (EFT) Practitioner and Retreat Facilitator, I am definitely no ordinary mentor and coach and I am sure my clients will agree with you on this.

Having mastered many various spiritual modalities and invested in my own personal growth since I was 17years of age, I have helped countless women throughout the world battle a range of personal and business challenges and overcome a string of limiting self-beliefs within themselves.

Many years ago, I felt trapped in an unrelenting cycle of anxiety, depression and constant negative thinking. I really struggled to find purpose in my then corporate sales career. When I finally found the courage to take a leap of faith and answer my soul's true calling, all elements of my life started to really feel like they were in alignment. I then started to experience success of a whole new magnitude, completely out of this world.

I have now set my sights on sharing my wisdom and supporting female spiritual entrepreneurs and leaders to experience the same incredible success and joy that I have been able to cultivate myself – by turning their budding business dreams into profitable, successful, loveable ventures. Putting to work my vast skill set and my many years of experience, I am so passionate about helping women learn how to own and use their gifts while earning a consistent income – it's what I was born to do! I feel it in my soul.

I am also so super passionate about helping women to create financial freedom and cultivate a healthy relationship with money and experience next level abundance so that they can be, do and have anything they desire in their life.

I am a rule breaker who has such a deep passion for living life on my terms and creating a life that fills my soul up every single day and I am here to give other women permission to do the same, and share their truth in their divine femine power.

Kat

Led by Soul

www.kathrynottobrino.com.au
Instagram: @kathrynottobrino
Facebook: kottobrino & kathryn.ottobrino.3

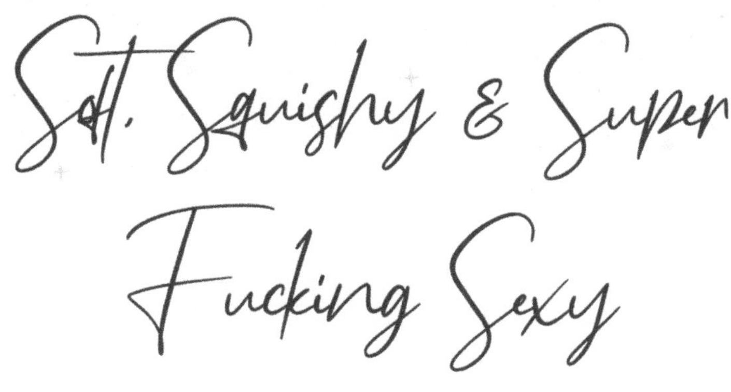

Soft, Squishy & Super Fucking Sexy

Kerry Mitchell-Bathgate

Sex, how fucking good is it!?

The pleasure it brings us, and the power we have over the men who want us. Whether we are big or small, short or tall, curvy or thin, men want us. Let me share my story on what I have learnt and why I am now a Soft and Squishy, Super Fucking Sexy Goddess.

Seventeen years ago, I was single, independent, carefree with lots of friends! I was working full-time, volunteering at a Community Radio station in the mornings and working weekends at a swingers club. I was busying living life, however I was insecure about myself, how I looked and the shape of my body. I was too fat, too short, not pretty enough – how could anyone find me attractive? Don't get me wrong, I was having lots of sex but I wasn't confident, and in turn, I was unhappy.

I met my (future) husband while I was working at the swingers club. It was love at first sight and eighteen months later we got married. I went from being a single, carefree thirty-three year-old to becoming a married woman with responsibilities, debts, plus a baby on the way! Although I was madly in love and happy, this was not what I had in mind for my life. I was going to have lots of girlfriends and boyfriends and I wasn't going to get married or have children. Instead, I was married for fourteen years, lived in four countries and had a beautiful, beautiful son who is a total dude, the light of my life and I love him to death!!

Fast forward to February 2019.

After ten years of travelling the world for my husband's work and a business we purchased in NZ, we came back to Perth and started to settle down.

I wasn't happy in my marriage and after living and working with my husband for the last four years, I needed to get away. I needed space to try and find myself, to be independent and free. I was able to get a FIFO (fly in fly out) job, which got me away from home and into a camp with hundreds of men! Before I started my new job though, I made sure that I had set up the house for my husband and son, as I was thinking of leaving. He had become more of a roommate than my husband over the years, and our sex life was non-existent.

I was extremely horny and very frustrated. The 'old Kerry' wanted to make a come back but I didn't know how! I did not have the confidence or the body, well I never had a body to start with and I was old! Forty-eight years old to be exact … who the hell would want to sleep with me!?!?!

The old Kerry was vibrant, sassy, loud, outrageous; and I so desperately wanted her back!

I had been working my FIFO job for a few swings and I was enjoying it. I was meeting new people, becoming more courageous, trying out some flirting techniques and slowing learning to 'like' me again.

My job had me changing to a new mine site and it was arranged that I would be picked up by a guy call Darren, who would drive me the three hours to my new location. Imagine my shock and delight when Darren turned out to be a very old friend I had lost contact with! For three hours we chatted, told our story of what we had been up to since we last saw each other, and then we both shared our sad story of sexual frustration within our marriages. About half way into the journey, he pulled over and I gave him a blow job. Oh the joy of sucking a hard cock again and the excitement of making him cum! Turns out sucking cock is like riding a bike, you never forget how! That night, we fucked our brains out! We were so comfortable with each other, we were able to just let go of our inhibitions and fuck until we were exhausted! Each night, after work, we would meet up in Darren's room, get naked, explore our desires and release our frustrations. Darren started to teach me, to show me I was desirable, that I was sexy, even with my soft and squishy curves! While we were catching our breath, we would talk about how nice it was to have each other on-site because it can be so lonely, and that no matter what ended up happening with us, we should always try to have a special friend on-site.

For two weeks, I had more sex than I had in fourteen years of marriage! I was feeling wonderful and alive. Glimpses of the 'old Kerry' were starting to return and I was happy. Darren was about to leave site for his one week RnR and we discussed how good we were both feeling and that we would pick up where we left off, when he returned to site.

Darren was killed in a car accident driving home from the airport.

I didn't find out about Darren until two days after the accident when the whole camp was told, and I was heartbroken. It wasn't until a few days later that I realised Darren had sent me a gift. He had sent me a new special friend.

Kent and I started talking the day Darren died. It was a simple conversation and then something happened. I can't explain it but something changed while we were chatting. One minute we were innocently talking and the next moment we were in his donga with him thrusting his cock down my throat. Kent was a well-hung, virile, thirty-four year old man who loved curvy older women!

Losing Darren rocked my world and made me realise that life is too short to be unhappy and sexually frustrated, so I asked my husband for an open marriage. I did not want to cheat on him, although I technically had, but wanted to be honest going forward. Surprisingly he said yes, so I went back to what I know and love best … a Swingers Club. Walking in was nerve-racking but as soon as I got through the door, I felt like I was home. More about the Club later.

I wasn't coping on-site with Darren gone, so I took on a temp job that moved me around different camps. I was on the front desk at one camp, when a fairly cute guy walked in to complain about his noisy neighbours. He gave me his room number and I looked it up on the system. I looked at his surname, 'Suckerdick,' looked at him and asked, "if it really is a good sucker," and he suggested I should find out for myself … which I did later that night!

It was the middle of the COVID-19 lock-down and all us ladies were rocking the 1800's look with hairy legs, due to the beauticians being closed. It was during this time that I discovered that men DON'T CARE if our legs are hairy!! Do you hear me girls … they don't care! Mr. Suckerdick (Tom) spent many evenings showing me just how turned on I made him, hairy legs and all, and it made me feel so very sexy!

I was feeler braver within myself, so I joined an Adults dating site that was linked to the Swingers Club. I was enjoying my rendezvous with the younger men on-site and thought I would see what young men were like in the 'real world.' I made no secret that I was an older woman, with lots of curves and that I was looking for a well-hung stallion with lots of stamina, in the 24-36 age bracket. Oh my Lord … the amount of men that replied was shocking and the quality of men was incredible!! So ladies, here is another thing I have learnt on my journey – men want older women, not girls. They want the curves and padding and most of all, they want a confident lady that will fuck them, as hard as they fuck you. They want you to moan and squeal and to tell them how hard you want it, or to scream when you are going to cum! They don't want a girl that doesn't want to ruin her hair or make-up or who just lays there, silent. Now I am an extremely loud woman, even with a pillow over my face, the neighbours will still hear me cum and I thought that was a turn-off to men, but no! So ladies, moan your heart out and tell your man exactly how you want him to fuck you!

The most memorable young man I had was a SAS soldier, who wanted to get a little bit rough with a MILF (remember Stifler's mom?), and I was happy to oblige. I had recently completed a BDSM 101 course and discovered that I'm not that kinky, I just love rough sex! Anyhow back to SAS Boy ... We chatted before I arrived and established the ground rules, (must wear a condom, no bruises above the neck or hair pulling from the roots, etc), so that when I arrived we just got straight to it. Do you know how hot it is to have a physically fit, young man want you the moment he opens the door?! Fuck, he was hard, very well-hung and fucking beautiful! I let him get as rough as he was comfortable with, and the sex was awesome! I also learnt a few things about my sexual psyche and how rough I actually like it.

SAS boy said he didn't want the younger girls (18-30) because they all thought they had to look and act like the porn models, perfect make-up and hair, too self-conscious, and they 'don't know how to suck cock properly.' Whereas, the older woman knows exactly what she wants, is confident in her body and isn't trying to get pregnant and marry you.

Are you seeing the pattern here ladies ...? I certainly was.

I started a new full-time job and was Perth based for around ten weeks, before heading back to site on a 3/1 (three weeks on, one week off) roster. Before I headed up to site, I had to go to the company's Perth warehouse to see supplies were available to take up to site. As I walked up the path to the warehouse, I saw this amazing man with a goatee, dressed in full PPE with a hard hat and safety glasses on, standing near the entrance of the warehouse, and all I wanted to do was go up and hug him!?!

WTF?!?

Hug him?

No seriously, the urge was incredibly strong and persistent and I was totally confused. I tried to compose myself and went to the counter and asked to see Mark, as he was going to show me around. Well guess who Mark was! The attraction was obviously mutual because within two minutes we were talking like long lost friends and expressing our weird and confused desire to hug each other. It was love at first sight for both of us.

I'm not backwards in coming forwards and was quite open about how I wanted to get him naked and do very naughty things to him, when he told me he was married. My heart sank as I said goodbye and walked away. However the chemistry between us was far too strong and we were making excuses to see each other on a daily basis. Yes, I knew he was married but the heart wants what the heart wants and oh my God, did I want him!!

The first time we had sex was like a scene out of high school! Even though he is married, he hadn't passionately kissed anyone in a very long time and he was so nervous kissing me! He was shaking as I dropped to my knees to pull down his pants and see his cock for the first time. I was able to see, every time we saw each other, the bulge in his pants, so I guessed he was well hung and I was not disappointed! His cock has a beautiful curve that was made especially for me. As I bent over his desk, he slid his perfect cock inside me and that curve hit all the right spots! Within a few strokes I was wetter than I had ever been, it was like his cock was made to fit perfectly inside me, and we came together, panting with exhilaration. We are made for each other, and although it might sound corny, he is my Soulmate. The chemistry between us is so powerful that even though we have tried to end it a few times, we simply can't.

Three weeks away from home is along time, but three weeks away from Mark felt like a lifetime! We spoke on the phone every morning, when he was driving to work and then every evening we were able to video chat for awhile. I would get naked, sit cross legged on my bed with my arms crossed over my belly, hiding it because I did not like my fat belly. Mark would 'tell me off' for doing that! He loves my belly, he loves how soft and squishy it is and didn't want me to hide it from him. I can tell you it took me awhile to be comfortable doing it, especially when you can see yourself on the screen but the constant compliments worked and now I LOVE my belly! We have been through a lot together and my belly is part of me, so of course I love her!

In the meantime, I had separated from my husband, our marriage was over but we remain very good friends and together we co-parent our son.

My confidence was continuing to grow, getting undressed in front of someone, with the lights on was no longer scary. The more confident I became, the sexier I was.

Let me say that again … the more confident I became, the sexier I was.

My social life was not coping with being away for three weeks at a time and I was beginning to miss Mark more each time I had to say goodbye, so I got a Perth based job. At the same time, Wayne, the Owner of the Swingers Club, called and asked if I was able to work Sundays for him. It would be 'hosting' the event, door work and running the bar, so I said yes without a seconds hesitation!

Anyone that knows me knows that I do not wear dresses. I am a jeans and black top sort of girl, with sneakers – no high heels! But after the first night working at the club, I started buying lingerie, sexy lacy bras and high heels! I was feeling so damn sexy I wanted to show off my curves! I brought little black dresses, with plunging necklines, so my beautiful cleavage could be seen.

My confidence at running the events on Sunday's are literally making me insatiable to men. They want to kiss me, touch me, bury their faces between my legs and taste me. They are feeding my confidence and in return I am feeling so damn sexy!

Who is this woman and where has she been for the last seventeen years?!

One thing I have always wanted to 'learn' to do is Squirt. I think it is so erotic, so hot because it is something you can't fake but I could never do it, until I met Sal. We were having a threesome one night and while I was sucking Paul's cock, Sal was fingering me. All of a sudden I squirted everywhere and yelled out with excitement!! Sal was very proud to tell me that he had read a book on how to make women squirt and I was the first he tried it on. I then got him to explain it and show me the technique, which Mark is becoming very good at now!!

I am not embarrassed to get naked at the club and let everyone watch, especially if I have a threesome with two big beautiful black men. The lust and passion I receive from men now is truly incredible and all because I have become so very confident about myself. My nickname is Gorgeous, and I most certainly am!

Mark has been very honest with me, he is not in a position to leave his wife and I have to accept that, although I hope, wish and pray that one day that will change. Mark also accepts me for who I am. He doesn't want me to change my lifestyle, so I am allowed to 'play.' Although it hurts him to know I am with other people, I will not commit to monogamy until he leaves his wife. The only condition is that I always use condoms (which I do) and if he asks, I tell the truth. However, the moment he leaves his wife, my playing days are over, but who knows when that will happen!

Now that I am so very confident in myself, I have decided to give stand-up comedy a go. I think I'm sort of funny because people laugh at my stories, but I never had the confidence before to get up on stage to try it. I have a 'prop' I am going to use and his name is George. (Google: 'I will love him and squeeze him and call him George'). George is a very large black dildo with a suction cap, that I bring out on Sunday at the Club and stick him to the bench. He is a great conversation starter and I think he will be a fantastic way to start my show by walking out on stage and sticking him to a table! Because my nickname is Gorgeous, I will call the show 'Gorgeous George'.

My six week comedy course starts soon but will be over by the time this book is released, so why not Google me and see if I'm living my comedy dream!

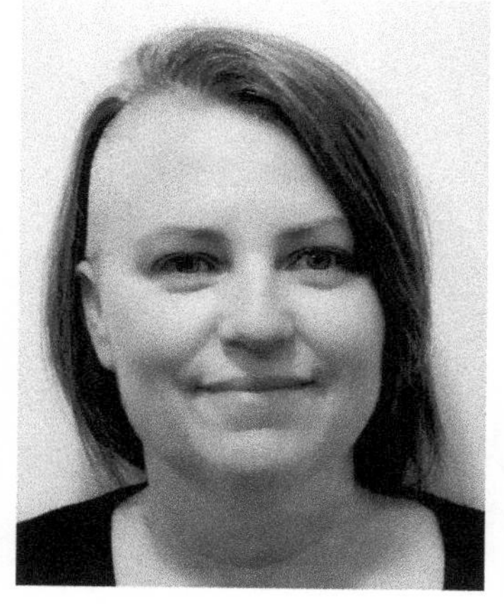

Kerry Mitchell-Bathgate

Hi, I'm Kerry Mitchell-Bathgate, well known for my loud, infectious laughing bubbly personality, I try to spread love and laughter wherever I go.

A fan of stand up comedy, I am preparing to go on stage and give this comedy thing a try with a good mix of sexual content and a big black dildo called George! (you'll read about George in my story)

A 49 year old lover of all things sexual, kinky and outrageous, sex and everything related to it, is my passion. Not afraid to speak of sex, I love to push the boundaries of peoples' comfort-zones. I want to empower my fellow sisters with the knowledge I have gathered and experienced, to talk openly about sex because every woman, everywhere, has a right to feel good about her own body and her sexuality.

I believe that no woman should ever be ashamed of her sexual experiences, needs or feelings and hope that women everywhere will realise that, if we are to be happy within our lives and relationships, our pleasure should always come first!!

I am Mum to a very cool 12 year old son, who is learning how to be a loving, caring boy while growing into an independent and self-sufficient young man.

Born and bred in Perth, I was introduced to international travel by my husband, when we moved to Canada in 2008, when I was 3 months pregnant. Liam was born in a beautiful part of Canada – St. John's, Newfoundland. We call him our Kanga-Newfie, which is as unique as Liam is.

After moving to Malaysia, Brisbane, back to Canada, Perth, Port Hedland and New Zealand, I am now settled back in Perth.

A self-confessed workaholic who gives everything to her job, I honesty enjoy working so much, I have a weekend job, working behind the bar of a Swingers Club, which means I get the best of both worlds – work and sex!

The Birthing Process

Kirsten Lyle

I tried really friggen hard to not make this chapter about birth, it seemed so cliché. I had another story in mind, but the words wouldn't come out onto the screen.

Literally at the eleventh hour my heart opened to the idea of actually writing about birth and the words started to pour. It makes sense. I am a Doula, I live for birth and when you think about it, birth is one of the very few things that connects us all.

We are ALL born.

Without the woman that stand in their power and surrender their body and souls, we, you and I wouldn't be here.

Birth connects and creates families and communities. It connects this life to the next and this lifetime to the next.

What is more powerful then connection? What is more powerful than creation?

So this isn't just going to be a chapter on how my kids where born but more on my experience with birth and how my own birth experiences have been the process for me to remember my purpose, and find my passion and power within to create. With that power I have been able to rebirth myself into a newer version who knows herself and her worth.

My first experience with birth, that I can remember, was while I was in my teens. We had purchased a horse from a rural station and within months of owning her it became pretty obvious she was in foal. Her body expanded, her breasts became engorged and her appetite increased dramatically. The signs that her body was preparing for birth became obvious. Her nipples become waxy, and one Saturday morning conveniently within daylight hours, we had a call from the woman we shared stables with that Sky was covered in sweat and breathing heavily.

I was with a friend at the time, so after a frantic call to my own mum, we made our way out to the stables. That sounds so posh and fancy, but realistically in Karratha the stables were a tin shed and a red dirt paddock surrounded by a fence. When we arrived, the word had got out to a few of the other horsey people, and we all stood around watching as my mare laboured on the ground. I could see she was working hard but I could also feel she was in distress. One of the women there had told us all to stay back, to not get in the way, but I could feel her drawing me in, so instinctually I went to her. I sat with her, stroked the front of her nose, and spoke softly to her. Her whole being relaxed in a second. It was pure magic. Soon after, her foal was born, and I moved back to make the space for her to clean and bond with him.

To say it was an incredible experience is an understatement. I had researched about how the birth process would go for her, but to be lucky enough to be there was amazing. It was raw and just happened. Nobody had to do anything. She cleaned him, and stood while the placenta or 'after birth' was born, the umbilical cord stopped pulsating and fell off and she nuzzled and pushed him to help him stand and then nurse. A whole new being was there right before our eyes; a not so tiny perfectly formed foal and just like that my mare was a mother. Everyone was elated and I decided right then when 'I grew up,' I was going to breed horses.

***

It was many years between that experience and the next, and in reality, the next time around was my time. I never wanted kids even though I was often told I was a natural-born mother. Babies and animals always hung out with me and my first ever job was babysitting our next-door neighbours' baby when I was twelve years old. Maternal was how I was described, but the desire to have my own was nil. I came from a broken family with a half-brother that was six years younger than me and really pissed me off in a lot of ways. I wouldn't say I enjoyed home life. I didn't know my dad, never got along with my stepdad, and didn't really have a great relationship with my mum. Therefore, to prevent 'fucking' my own kids up, I just wouldn't have any. Then my best friend had a baby. Fuck, it was like a switch flicked on inside of me, and all I could think about was having a baby. My partner and I had spoken about it but nothing serious, but once I made my decision, I just told him I was ready and that was that.

Everyone talks about the glowing, beautiful experience that is pregnancy but that wasn't the case for me. Nausea all day every day; I would vomit at the smell of EVERYTHING. Hell, I would vomit if we walked past dog shit even if it had no smell. It was beyond a joke and didn't help with the fatigue. I was emotional, of course, but I also struggled with the changes to my body. I didn't feel beautiful, in fact, I felt like a fat whale, and our maternity system didn't help with that.

I wanted to birth at home; well we were living with my stepdad while waiting for the titles to our block, but you know 'home.' I still held trust in the process from watching my horse. I knew I would gravitate towards water and I didn't really see why I would want pain relief. But I lived in a dead zone between two publicly funded homebirth services and neither serviced my area. I didn't know that privately-practising midwives were a thing back then, so I rang my local hospital and they booked me into the midwifery group practise. I was kicked out of the MGP at around twenty weeks 'in case my weight increased too much,' even though I was losing weight from the constant vomiting. Go figure. My only choice now was to book in with a private obstetrician, a service that was a lot different to the homebirth I had hoped for.

A great friend held me a baby shower and we did a belly cast that I later destroyed because I hated the way it looked. I felt like a vessel, and I even remember describing being pregnant as living with a huge parasite. I had no idea that all the challenges I was going through emotionally and spiritually were all a part of the process; the parts of becoming a mother that happen long before the babe is born. Matrescence.

Her birth was much like my pregnancy; I was not in control. I really thought if I had read everything and gathered all the information, it would ensure the birth would go exactly as I planned, but once I stepped foot into that hospital, the system took control. I was coerced into procedures I didn't want, that I still now don't understand why were performed and even had things done that I did not give consent to at all.

I went from my waters breaking on their own and labouring in a room with only my partner. Managing the surges with my breath and movement for around 3 hours until someone remembered us and realised, I was 7 cm's dilated. To a birth suite with a midwife my partner is sure was drinking whiskey in the back room, flat on my back not allowed to move. I was hooked up to every fucking devise possible, cannular, bp cuff, heart rate monitor, ctg and even the syntocin drip that's used to speed labour up. Um wtf? My heart rate was high, well derh, so I was stabbed with a dose of pethidine that I didn't want to help relax me. I had my babe sucked out of me with the ventouse while I was off with the fucking fairies.

So yeah, I had a healthy baby, coz you know that's what everyone tells you is important, but I walked away seriously emotionally traumatised. She was beautiful but I was broken and had lost all trust in my body, and that was exasperated by my milk never 'coming in.' That birth affected everything. My body is a fairly obvious one, though everything healed reasonably quickly. My relationship, not just because of the usually sleep deprivation and adjustments from 2-3 people at home, but because of what I was processing. I have the most vivid memory of standing in the shower when I was around three months postpartum. I was ugly crying. I tried to only do that in the shower so I could 'hide' it. My partner came in and asked me why I was crying. I had no way to tell him what I was going through. I have always been great at feeling, but expressing those feelings in words is sometimes a real struggle. All I could come out with was, 'it wasn't the way it was supposed to be.' Of course, he couldn't understand the depth that simple statement meant. There was nothing he could 'fix,' nothing he could change, and so eventually he would just leave me alone in my grief. Because that's what it was.

Sex was also an issue after birth. No matter what position we tried it was uncomfortable. No matter how much lube we used, it hurt. It pulled and felt tight at the opening to my vagina. It was like there was now skin where there was no skin before and it was not flexible. I can only put this down to the way I was stitched after I tore to my arsehole. When you tell someone, they are hurting you every time they are intimate with you, it gets to a point where they feel you are just not interested, and so our sex life dried up. On the odd occasion we did have sex I didn't enjoy it. I was in pain but being in pain and connecting with my partner was better than not connecting at all. I honestly don't know why I never went to a doctor to be checked out. I guess I took it as the new normal.

***

It was my daughter's first birthday party when I realised I was pregnant again. All the same symptoms started arriving; super sore boobs, nausea and vomiting, fatigue, the fucking nightmares, heartburn bleh. We discovered at our nine-week dating ultrasound it was twins! Wait what? Two? No way! My bestie and I had only just been joking about having twins and me being a smart arse, I said I would ask them to take one out if that was the case. My partner was ridiculously excited and was ringing people before the ultrasound was over, while I lay there silently mortified.

I became the perfect patient through this pregnancy. I was traveling up to the expert maternity hospital an hour away for appointments because you know, twins were too high a risk to be born vaginally at my local. I felt very fortunate that I stayed pregnant to term with the babies. Everyone told me they would be early. Basically, the fear of all the things that could go wrong was laid out to me at every step of the way just because there were two babies in my belly.

At thirty-eight weeks I chose to be induced. I was done.

I was heavily advised to have an epidural put in place because twin #2 was breech. My waters were broken and the induction went smoothly. My midwives were lovely, I didn't feel much at all and I didn't get left alone, not even for a minute. A vastly different experience right there. When it came time to push twin #1's heart rate dropped low and we were rushed off to theatre. By the time we got in there and I was prepped for surgery, his heart rate had calmed and I managed to push him out of my vagina! Woo, nice work. He went over to the little cot thingo and it was time to birth twin #2. Yeah, she is a stubborn one. Now that she had all the room in the womb she had turned and was laying on her side. After almost half an hour of watching the ultrasound machine showing the doctor's hand inside of my belly trying to grab either her head or her legs, the call was made that she was coming out the sunroof. By that time, I didn't give a shit and was just relieved that it would all be over.

I spent over a week in hospital after the twins were born. During that time, we were evacuated because of a fire, walking down what felt like 50 flights of stairs holding a newborn is not easy two days after a caesarean. Thank fuck my husband, Andrew was there at the time to carry the other baby. My milk still took a week to come in, even after tandem feeding and pumping between feeds, but when it did it was like the floodgates had opened haha. There was definitely an abundance.

Taking two babies' home to a twenty-month-old was an absolute challenge. Her behaviour changed, our relationship changed, and we all fell into a routine that felt necessary, but did not align to my parenting wishes at all. I'm not going to lie, it was a struggle, but overall I felt like the whole experience was a lot more positive. I called the shots. I made the final decision. It was by no means wonderful, but it surpassed my very little expectations. And as a bonus, sex didn't hurt anymore! Giving birth vaginally again must have stretched the tight skin back out to where it belonged.

***

Our final babe was born six years later. In our lounge room into water, surrounded by his siblings, a privately-practising midwife that we had known the whole way through the pregnancy, a beautiful friend that took on the role of my doula, and our pets. When they say midwifery care is the gold standard of maternity care they aren't joking. Seeing the same person for every appointment, building the relationship up over time, is amazing. This person becomes a friend, a confidante, they know you, your body and what is normal for you.

This seriously made the world of difference during this pregnancy. I was honoured. Not just the baby that I held in my womb, but me, the person, the mother to be was held and honoured in all the messy emotions, though all the ups and downs, through good times and bad. Every decision that needed to be made came with a conversation about not just the risks, but the benefits and alternatives as well, and there was never ever any pressure to make a decision on that day.

It was seriously amazing. It was exactly the 'way it was meant to be' I was referring to while ugly crying in the shower. It was a whole process leading up to and following the day I gave birth, not just the day the baby was born but the day I gave birth. The day I became a mother again. Just putting it like that still gives me goosebumps. It puts the focus back on me, the person that grew and birthed and surrendered so many things to bring this new life to this earth. I held importance in this experience, I wasn't just the vessel.

The whole experience felt so new but so perfectly ancient all at the same time. It took me back to a time were women were celebrated, where we lived in community and revered the birthing process. It brought trust back to my body, to my intuition, to my instinct. It felt sacred. It was a rite of passage. It truly highlighted how transformational that time is and how it has lasting effects on our physical, mental, and spiritual beings. It made me question why it was only just now, after my third pregnancy, I was feeling this way. Every woman deserves to feel like this after they have walked this path. Every birthing person should know the power they hold in their womb space of creation and know the feeling of reverence along that journey.

It was then I realised I was never going to breed horses, I needed to be in the birth space with birthing humans! I needed women to walk away with more than a healthy baby. So I took the first steps to work as a doula. Since then I have seen powerful women roar and sing and dance and sway as they birth their babies. I have cried and laughed, stood back, and held space and literally held women up while they birth their babies. I have felt the moment babes soul enters their body and they choose the moment they want to be born, and every single time I walk away a different person. Every single time I hold those women and their partners in the utmost respect. Every time I am reminded of the power within them and the power within me.

I once heard doulas being described as the 'energetic portal holder's', of the birth space and god that makes my juices flow. That is exactly how I see my role. My role in your journey is to bring back the reverence, the ceremony and to help facilitate that dream state in birth. The state that's often referred to as 'labour land.' To hold, be present with you and guide you if needed as your consciousness travels to any level it needs, to bring your babe into this world.

I am a guide. I am a guardian. I am a gate-keeper.

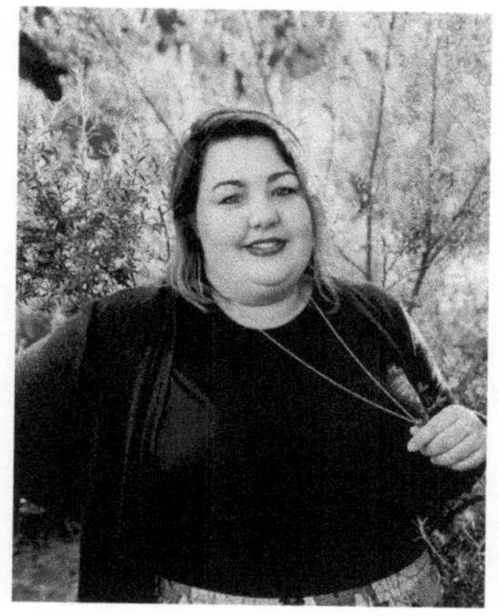

Kirsten Lyle

Howdie, I'm Kirsten Lyle, Impassioned advocate of birthing rights. Now published author, Starseed, Light worker, Ceremony holder and owner of Kirsten Lyle – Full Circle Doula.

My soul's work is nourishing people transitioning through pivotal times in their lives, while also creating ceremony around sacred rites of passage including menarche, matressence, birth and death.

I am 36 years old and living on Pinjarup country (Pinjarra) in Western Australia. I grew up on Jaburrara country in the Pilbara spending a lot of my time camping, exploring the bush land near our home, riding my horse, reef walking while the tides were low and out on the boat fishing and snorkelling. I still feel a strong connection to that land and it's often still the setting of my dreams.

Once I finished my high schooling in 2001, I went on to do a floristry apprenticeship and worked in the local florist until I moved down south and bummed around at the beach for close to a year, until I started work in the kitchen of the local hospital. I learnt a lot about life and death while working in that place.

I am a wife and a mother of four children that each teach me continuing lessons on the importance of coming together in circle and ceremony and the ways in which we can combine parenting and sacred celebration.

It's these lessons and experiences that I bring with me whenever I am in the birth or death space.

Experiencing the coming and going of souls to and from this earthly plane, through the energetic portals in these spaces, is always a profound experience and one I hold in deep respect each and every time.

My energy work offers a loving embrace that reminds your body and spirit they are capable of releasing what no longer serves you and heal on a soulful level. My guidance is honest, heartfelt and without bias or judgment.

Reverence from first to last breath x

www.kirstenlyle.com.au
Instagram: @kirstenlyle_fullcircledoula

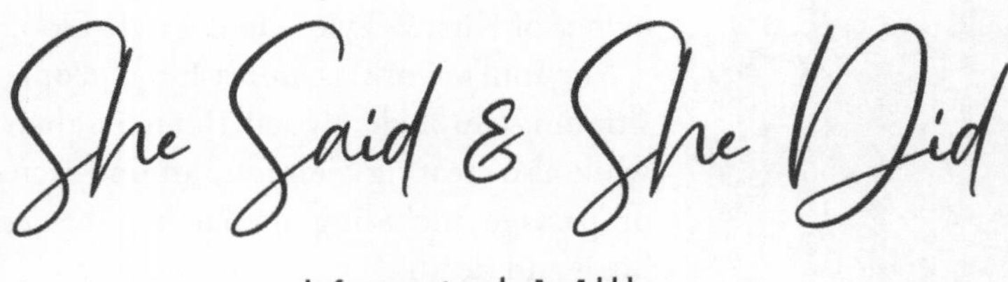

She Said & She Did

Krystal Miller

"She said it softly
She said it loudly
She screamed it. Still no one heard.

She's too meek
She's too obvious
She's too in-your-face. Still no one believed her.

She didn't speak.
She didn't whisper.
She didnt show her pain. No one saw it coming."

TRIGGER warning. If you have read the other incredible women's chapters, then you know that some contain experiences that may be triggering. If you are feeling overwhelmed, please be kind to yourself and ensure you take the time to heal.

My chapter may contain a bit of swearing and fuckery, so please be warned! I like to think of it as a combination of horror and humour!

Much love.

My earliest memories are filled with traumatic experiences, with all the subtle ways I had been dismissed, squashed, lessened, manipulated, and/or broken.

You wouldn't know by looking at me now. You wouldn't know by *knowing* me now; I was once, very much a victim. I try to present myself well – 'Look good, feel good' has been my motto. I've always tried to hide from my pain by ensuring my reflection did not show the true depth of it. It's not just the way I dress or present myself, it's also my - no bullshit, assertive, (sometimes fake) confidence.

But here I am now, feverishly typing away in bed, with my third baby girl sleeping soundly next to me. She's five months old and I see my reflection in her smile. I also smile a lot; it's my resting face. You may think I'm an optimist, I'm not; I'm a realist.

My story is not unlike many other women's; I was a victim of sexual and mental abuse as a child. There is a cycle of abuse that has continued throughout history in my family. My abuser was not blood-related, but he played a pivotal role in my life. He took a lot from me and tried to fuck with my head. He almost succeeded, until my twenty-first birthday, where I took my power back. That night, I became me.

Perfectly, imperfect me.

I was a fourteen year-old girl when I ran away from home, and my abuser. The last straw for me was while cutting bread for dinner. He came up behind me and kneed me so hard I was sure he'd broken my coccyx.

I stood there, a knife in my hands, shaking and using every ounce of my being not to turn around and stab him with it. I slammed it down, and ran out screaming, 'I fucking hate you!' as I jumped the fence.

That was the last time I lived at home.

I'd never been a 'normal' kid. I was always told to be quiet, stop talking, stop asking so many questions, stop listening in on other people's conversations, no you don't need to know why, 'why can't you be like [any other random name!]? You are just too much, Krystal …'

Those things became my mother-fucking super powers!!! Before that, questioning 'why' to everything was my path to destruction!

We've all been there, laying in bed, feeling sorry for ourselves, wondering what we did wrong or why us and not them?

I know this part of introducing myself to you is going to sound like a big fat victim sesh, but I've got to lay some foundations! You have to know how shitty things can be, so you can see how epic the good shit is!

The night I ran away was the start of some pretty horrific stuff; some poor choices were made.

Yep, I was that girl, looking for love in all the wrong places. I lost my virginity that night to a boy who saw an opportunity, and took it.

In the two weeks after jumping the fence, I got very sick and lost ten kilos. I'm sure that living off 2-minute noodles was not doing me any favours, but it turned out it was most likely caused by the stress-induced disease that was rotting away my insides!

Crohn's Disease.

Crohn's Disease is an auto-immune disease eats away at the lining and the fatty tissue of your intestines, causing ulceration and agony. It's like living with the worst case of Gastro 24/7 - on your period.

Geez, how much worse can this story get, right?!!!

Finally getting diagnosed was a fuckery of all fuckeries. Small country town, with small country town minds, I was dismissed as being an attention whore; or maybe just a whore.

I'd been living in a youth homeless shelter, and after six months I'd finally found a flat that I could rent. I tried to continue to go to high school but it was impossible. I was sleeping twenty-two hours a day, waking to go to school on the bus, only to have to turn around and go back to bed.

My body didn't want to play the game, and my mind was also up for self-destruction and torment. Every moment of waking time, I'd replay everything anyone had ever criticised me for. Everyone else's life looked so much better than mine, and I couldn't understand why I was being punished. What had I done to deserve loneliness and pain?!

Wasn't I a good person? Didn't I try to make people feel good? Wasn't I loving enough? I knew I did not deserve to be abused by anyone.

Watch this bitch flip the script though!

After years of the same bullshit, a few momentous moments of growth and power saw me change the dialogue in my brain. Instead of miserably asking those questions, they became more like; Why the fuck aren't I good enough?!!! I am! I am a good person. I am deserving,!

At this point, I was so sick I was constantly shitting myself and basically a twenty-one year-old reclusive nun. I'd been to hell and back. I still wore the emotional scars from the sexual abuse, but even more so the mental.

One thing I've realised over time is that predators innately know who is the perfect prey. I was just that; desperate to be loved by a father figure, and desperate enough to be manipulated and gaslighted. Even after I ran away, I kept quiet. I had to tell some people, but fourteen year-old me thought everyone would be better off without me. 'Out of sight, out of mind.' My self-worth had been taken from me. My mind had been fucked. He continued to act as if nothing had happened; that it was all in my head, and would walk around town as if he were being victimised by my 'bullshit' accusations.

All this time, my mum was stuck between the unknown and potential hearsay as to why I'd left. I couldn't bear to face her and tell the truth. I thought it would hurt her. I loved my mum so much, I didn't want to ruin her life with my trauma. She'd always told me, no matter what, I could tell her anything, but I just couldn't do it. I didn't appreciate at the time that what I was doing was far worse.

Fucking fourteen year-olds, hey?!!

My mum finally left him, and eventually met an incredible man I am proud to call Dad. He is everything to me and I'm beyond grateful for the love he gives my mum and to me, and my family. He will always be my MacGiver! I don't know where I'd be without the love and support of my parents. I love you guys! The tough times have brought us closer and I am so grateful.

Anyways, back on track …

Although I've had some pretty shitty times in my life, I am lucky my mum raised me, on her own, to have a good, solid foundation and good morals. I've also had some incredible influences who have contributed to me becoming the fierce woman I am today, so a massive shout-out to all those epic women!

One of the pivotal moments towards redefining and rediscovering my worth, was the moment I decided to become a topless barmaid. Oh My God! You did what, Krystal?!!

Yep, I was a topless barmaid. Before you jump on the horror train, let me break some shit down for you. Absofuckinglutely, there are girls and women who do this for some pretty terrible reasons, but I wanted to do this - for my mental health. Once again, you are probably horrified right?!

Think about it this way; my body and my sexuality was taken from me. The first abuser was just that, my first, and because of him I was an easy target. Working as a topless barmaid was my way of safely reclaiming back my body and my sexuality. It was on my terms and I had the power and was safe behind the bar.

I learnt about myself and men. I found 'me' in all that twisted therapy!

A few years later, at twenty-one, I was no longer a victim or a possession to be had. It was my twenty-first birthday and my friends and I went to the local pub. All of a sudden, like a predator stalking me; through the sea of people dancing he came up to me. He'd become cocky and with suppressed honesty and a slippery tongue, told me how amazing my tits looked in my dress and how he loved touching them(when I was younger).

Child Krystal and empowered Krystal took to battle in my mind. For a moment all I wanted to do was cave into myself, but somehow a fire lit inside me. The anger boiled up and all the ways I had been gaslighted, manipulated and abused, spilled out. I screamed at him and made my next big step to becoming a strong fierce woman who lived in her power, wholly and solely.

I took away that motherfuckers power over me and called him a disgusting paedophile who had no right to touch me or talk to me!!!

Phew! Anyone else need to take in a deep breath too?! Stay with me gorgeous.

Holy shit, twenty-one was a big fucker of a year! It was the same time that my Gastroenterologist told me, 'It's time;' to cut the disease out and fit me with an ostomy.

Cutting out the diseased part of my bowel meant that I would now need a bag where all my bodily waste (aka shit), would go. He wasn't convinced I would cope. In hindsight, he probably was a genius and knew how to use one's stubbornness against them! Smart man because I was like; Bitch, hold my beer! Watch me be all coping and shit!

Those nightly spins around the ol' block of self-destruction were not going to work on me anymore! Jesus, I was taking the wheel!

Surgery removed six kilograms of diseased bowel, along with my asshole; technical term, anus.

Ohhh I've got you intrigued now haven't I?! No asshole? Nope, unless we're including my hubby!

I took this surgery to be a blessing. I was to be disease free, even if it wasn't forever, but it was going to give me a moment and an opportunity;. to weed out all the assholes from my life, literally and figuratively.

So, I'd have to poo into a bag! Anything was going to be better than the non-living I was doing at the time. Crohns was killing me slowly and I could feel its poison coursing through me, eating me alive.

I am pleased to announce that my surgery was a success and yes, all the assholes left the building!

Did I care? Of course I did? Why? Because even as strong as I was, I was convinced I'd never find someone who would love me.

Relationships with people, intimate or not, have always been hard for me. I can give you all of me, but I'm not so good at being vulnerable.

I've always loved with my whole heart and soul. I've been told too often that I give my all too quickly, and boy, has that bitten me on the ass many times. But that is how I love and I don't know any other way.

Loving others and not receiving the same back can be heartbreakingly insightful. I learnt a valuable lesson. It's not about how much you love someone, but how much they love YOU.

That doesn't necessarily make a person an asshole. Mis-compatablitiy doesn't make someone an asshole, it just makes you mismatched, and that's okay!

It's okay to end a relationship. It's okay to walk away if it doesn't feel right. We, as a society, need to stop teaching and spreading lies about attraction being about proving yourself worthy!

If you stop and look, it's incredible how moments in time can define you. Moments of hardship and torture can shape and polish who you are - if you let them. Or are you stuck in the same rut? Do things continually keep happening in your life and you just can't seem to break the cycle? I'm sure we've all been there, it's something we've all experienced. But I want to give you something that has truly been valuable for me in my life: You are destined to repeat the same mistakes, until you have learnt the lesson you were destined to learn. You cannot move forward in life if you continue to cycle through the same bad choices with the same mentality.

Every lesson has been hard. Some lessons have been all consuming and I'm honestly not sure how I am still here today. Maybe it's because I know fundamentally that horrible moments don't last forever. There are always options, and when they do pop up, you just have to take them.

Being sick and fucking a lot of shit up along the way has left me feeling like I'm drowning at times, but I never apologise for crying or being honest about how I feel.

I allow myself to wallow. I sit in my misery as long as I fuckingwellneed to! Cause Holy Shit I've deserved it. We all need permission for that moment to be as self-pitying as we need to be.

BUT

Get back up. Remember that while we need to be in that moment of pity and tears, life will keep going and we will need to pick ourselves up - eventually.

It's the tough times that have shaped me into the woman I am today. They can call me what they want. They can put me into a box. They can try to tell me who I am, but I know who I am and I am comfortable with my shadow.

So here I type as a thirty-seven year-old woman, now married with three gorgeous, crazy kids! I never expected my life to be like this. My husband is the biggest pain in my ass but who says marriage is easy? I'm joking. He is great, has a wonderful soul and a laugh that is contagious. He stands by my side and has accepted every flaw and seen me as beautiful. I am very grateful for him and the life that we have built together.

I met him at a time when I was jaded and wasn't going to play society's games anymore. If I wanted to hold his hand, I was going to. I said it completely honestly and it worked for him. Almost eleven years later, here we are!

Life isn't easy. Health and trauma can rear their ugly head occasionally, but I'm a stubborn shit who refuses to be told what to do. As a young girl, I wasn't given control of my body or my disease, so today I'm a control freak. Don't get me wrong, I love chaos, as long as I'm in control of it!

I am a huge fan of Counselling and it has often helped me with my trauma but there are many other unique modes of self-therapy too.

I have many tattoos and piercings now. They're moments in time with significant meaning. They've helped me to redefine pain into pretty artwork. The lion on my stomach covers scars and represents being fierce, loyal, and proud but elegant. The 3 butterflies on my side with the Greek words, Νέα ζωή mean New

Life, for my three year anniversary of my first surgery. The pocket watch and flowers along my thigh mark the time of birth for my beautiful first born. Next to that is the elephant who represents my second. The two roses above my knee are for the twins we lost in 2018. On my side, I have the picture my husband drew of us as stick people, but I threaten him regularly that if he pisses me off I'll just add another stick person and it will look like the 3 kids instead! Haha.

I have a few more planned; one being my sleeve which is a vintage ship battling through stormy water, and the quote, 'the pessimist complains about the wind, the optimist expects it to change and the realist adjusts the sails.'. That is my life's motto. And of course, I need to find something to represent my newest babe!

My love for my husband was unexpected. My besty still laughs because she'd always reassure me that I would find someone and have babies, even when I would cry that I'd never have children. I was told at fifteen that I would be very lucky to have children because of my disease, and I believed them.

I was so desperate to grow up and be a wife and mother, but I was convinced I wouldn't ever be that lucky. How hilarious that reality is so much harsher! I mean, don't get me wrong! I've got my dream but damn, it's hard sometimes!

After my surgery at twenty-one, I moved to Greece and lived there for three years. I was in love with a Greek man who will always hold a special place in my heart. He showed me love despite my constant insecurities and never cared about my Ostomy bag! He'd even jump into the shower with me without my bag on! It was with him I learnt to accept love and feel deserving of it.

We tried for a long time to have a baby but it wasn't to be and when we did fall pregnant, we lost the baby. Eventually our relationship broke down; the cultural differences and living so far from home, took its toll. I moved back to Australia and left behind the most incredible friends who had become my family.

Everything happens for a reason. A few months after returning to South Australia, I got a job and was sent to Darwin to work for sixteen weeks. It was there I met my husband.

If you ask him about the first time we met, he describes me as 'this woman walking into the morning briefing with both hands bandaged (damn arthritis!), tongue out and making wanking gestures with her hand!' He also says that I have upside down eyes! Jerk! Haha!

I noticed him, the same day. He was team leader and had thick curly blonde locks poking from his cap that made him look like Dicky Knee, a puppet from the popular TV show, Hey! Hey! It's Saturday!

We walked into the office and he sat down, took his shoes and socks off and put his feet up on the desk. I thought, 'who the fuck is this dickhead?'

But he was hilarious, kind, gentle and we got along like a house on fire! He called me "little fella" and we made plans to go fishing on his boat. That didn't happen, but he did take me on a date to see Jackass 3D and the next day to the local museum. I was impressed and nervous! We spent the whole time talking and it was just so easy.

He didn't know about my Ostomy bag and I wasn't sure I would tell him straight away. I told him on the third date, and his response was epically him to a T. He didn't care but asked if everything else still worked!

I'd told him from our very first date that I would not be having sex with him, so he didn't make any moves at all. By our third date I was annoyed that he hadn't even tried to kiss me! Dude, I'm only here for a few weeks! A girls got needs too and I only meant I wouldn't be having sex on the first date! I had to set some boundaries!

Third date, I made the move. I pushed him down on the couch and kissed him. And the rest is history!

Three months later, I moved back to SA. We'd agreed to stay in touch because we liked each other but I was stubborn and jaded - I was not moving for a man! Oh silly Krystal! Turns out that despite using contraception, BAM! I was pregnant. What a beautiful surprise! Especially after being told that I couldn't have kids!

Telling him over the phone was my only option. That's not how I wanted to do it. I sat with the news for eight days before I couldn't hold in the secret any longer. Anyone who knows me, knows that I can keep someone else's secret but I cannot hold my own!

I apologised for not giving him a choice but I would be keeping the baby. He had the choice of what role he'd play in our lives. I would have respected any choice, but I really liked him so I hoped he would pick us. He just had to clarify that it was his first! Haha.

Four months later, I moved back to Darwin to start a life together. We both really liked each other and were lucky to grow to love each other alongside me being pregnant, not because we were pregnant.

It's not been an easy ride, and boy, has our relationship had some pretty epic testing. When our baby was born, my bowel perforated and I became septic. No one would believe me at the hospital and I became weak and disempowered. I almost died.

His family flew me, and our 6 month old, to Perth, Western Australia where they discovered I had two 5cm abscesses full of fecal matter and puss floating around in my abdomen. My body was shutting down, I was forced to stop breastfeeding, could not hold my baby and was hospitalised for a month. I was having forty-two degree temperatures and fits. I needed more surgery to clean me out and remove another small portion of my bowel.

I was terrified. I was terrified for my baby. I didn't want my baby to grow up without a mama. Though I don't remember much of that time, my body has retained the trauma so significantly it's a part of my DNA. Writing this I feel my body tighten and my pulse quicken.

Luckily I recovered, but the stress on me, and my baby daddy's way of dealing with it, didn't match up. He lived in denial and I so desperately needed a rock and someone to hold my hand,- if only just to have him understand my pain

I love him but also hated him for the way he dealt with it. I felt alone and so scared. Counselling saved us. . When I recovered, we went for walks along the beach and would talk honestly about everything. We grew back together.

Our second babe didn't come so easily. 2.5 years of trying and fertility treatment finally gave her to us. Our third was just as big a surprise as the first!

Marriage Counselling and even just Counselling for yourself is so important. We see it more like a marriage tune up or service. Sometimes we're good and sometimes I want to choke him in his sleep!

Reflecting, it's easy to wish you knew the stuff you know now back then. But I am proud of who I am today. Even on my dark days, I have no regrets. I am who I am, I cannot change and will not change because I know that fundamentally I am a good person and try every day to do the best I can.

So this is for everyone in the world who's felt suppressed, alone & insecure.

When you're feeling like you can't fit into their square hole. When you've tried suppressing, and shaving off your sides to fit but somehow it's just never enough.

When you've grown up knowing that their bullying and criticism of who you are, what you look like and what you do, just isn't right.

This is for you.

Today I'm going to lead you and show you another dimension …

Here are a range of holes. They're all made to be flexible and mould around who you are at every stage of your life.

You have permission.

Permission to *ignore them* shouting out at you, hoping to bring you down and to keep you feeling like you don't fit.

You don't have to be down there. You have choices.

You don't have to believe anything they say. You don't have to make it your truth. Listen to your gut (instincts) and let that lead the way.

If something makes YOU happy and someone comes along trying to deflate you or chip away at you, I want you to ask yourself, 'does their opinion really matter or define me?'

I don't want to be one of the sheep. I don't want to be 'normal,' whatever that is.

I want to be whoever, and whatever I feel in the moment. I want to grow. I want to be kind. I want to empower. I want you to be completely, totally, unapologetically …

YOU.

BE THE BEST VERSION of you.

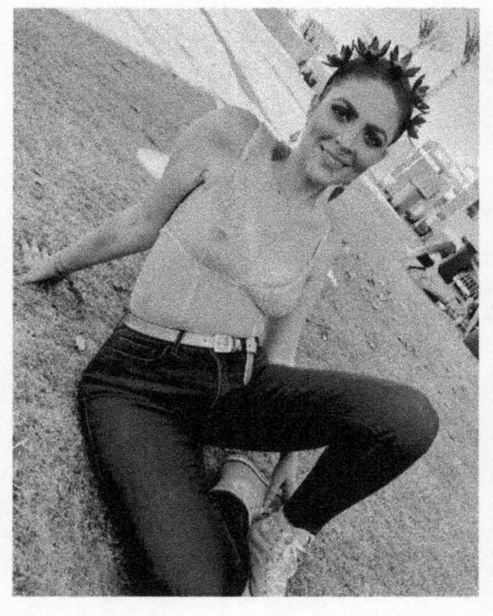

Krystal Miller

So who am I? Writing a bio is hard for me. I'm many things wrapped up in many experiences both good and bad. I'm not just a wife, a mother, a daughter, an aunt, a friend or a blogger. I'm all of those things and yet I'm not defined by one single one of them.

I am just me.

A woman who somehow has managed to wake up every morning and is grateful for every moment she is still here. A bit of a gypsy who has found it hard to settle in one place but has enjoyed every moment, including living in Greece for 3 years.

I express myself through writing, clothes and the colour of my hair! I enjoy messing with people's expectations or stereotypes!

Generally, I'm just a foulmouthed mama who is like everyone else, just trying to get the kids to school on time, keep them clean and raise them with good morals and foundations! What you see is what you get with me 24/7 and I try to find the time to write, inspire and empower others. Most of the time inspiration only comes to me when i'm in the shower and my phone isn't near me!

Diagnosed with Crohn's Disease at 14 years old after running away from a traumatic childhood, I always thought that the powers that be must have made this happen so that I could help others through writing a book and here we are! I think we all look to find a reason to justify and explain the reasons that bad things happen in our lives.

I'm a Bag Lady - not the homeless kind - just out there trying to rid the world of all the assholes, the metaphorical and physical!

So you may have already guessed, but I swear - a lot.

Life has been pretty awful at times, but I do my best to be both humorous and realistic.

I am raw, honest and straight to the point with a huge dollop of humorous smartass. I believe in being completely authentically yourself, raw and unapologetic, so long as you're still being a decent human! After having my second baby in 2015, I started a blog called Bag Lady Mama. I wanted to help empower women after experiencing a life time of pigeonholing and disempowerment

Life is about living it to the fullest with your heart full.

www.bagladymama.com
Instagram: @bagladymama
Facebook: bagladymama

My Ladybits are Lemons

Lisa Johnson

I was born to be a mum. I knew it. Everyone knew it, right from when I was thirteen and used to help my seventeen year-old sister with her new bub. It was the most natural thing in the world to me. I had my life planned. Get engaged at eighteen, married at twenty and have my first bub by twenty-one.

The problem was that at nineteen I still did not get a period and every year I would ask my mum why and she would tell me she was a late starter, so I probably was too. That worked for a couple of years, but then my mum, who worked at King Edward Women's hospital got talking to a specialist one day and he suggested I go in for tests. So I did, and life changed from that moment on.

After several long and invasive tests I was diagnosed with Turners Syndrome (Mosaic), which is a chromosome disorder that has a lot of different variations. Mine included having only one ovary and it was a streak ovary, meaning it had no tissue and eggs. I also had a small uterus, so even if by some miracle I fell pregnant, I would be bedridden for the last three months of a pregnancy -which I would have been okay with if there was TV, a good book and chocolate! My very old specialist, with a cold factual bedside manner, informed me that I would never have children.

Hold up, somebody forgot to tell our creator that I needed ovaries and a hospitable womb, but instead I got served lemons! Lemons, instead of the crucial lady bits I needed to fulfil my dreams.

Let me tell you, if I had shares in Kleenex I would have made a fortune. What will I do with my life? I would never get married or have kids. Who would want someone who wasn't perfect, who couldn't give them a mini version of themselves to play footy with or go to netball with. No man would want a woman who couldn't produce the goods. Life was never going to be what I had grown up wanting. I was going to be a lonely old spinster cat- lady at nineteen years old.

Then when I was twenty, I met my now husband. In my opinion he was rock star gorgeous (I still think that now when I look at his fifty-three-year-old face). I couldn't believe he wasn't already snatched up. I couldn't believe this handsome man wanted to be with me. So I took the opportunity and ran with it. I put him on the highest pedestal and thought I was the luckiest girl alive. I remember getting ready for our second date. I was standing in the bathroom putting my face on, wearing a short nightie. He was checking out my pins (back then they were pretty good) and I looked at him and said, 'Just in case this gets serious, you need to know I can't have babies.'

I'm not sure if he was confused, shocked or bloody terrified about a statement that contained the word babies on a second date, when his only thought was probably getting a beer and getting laid! Surprisingly though, there was still a third date, a fourth and a fifth. A couple of years later, when he said he wanted to discuss something serious with me, my immediate thought was that he was going to end it with me, because being a bit older now he probably realised he wanted a real woman, a whole woman, a woman who could give him a family. I nearly jumped in first and called it because I thought it would be easier for him if I did, but I'm so glad I didn't. Instead, after a drawn out conversation to get around to his question, he told me that, at only twenty-three he wasn't sure if he wanted kids, but was sure that he loved me and wanted to spend his life with me. He proposed, I cried and thirty-two years later we are still going strong. Yes we've had some ups and downs, some sad, some testing times in our life, but right now I probably love him more now than I did then, in a more mature and equal way. Once, I had him on a pedestal and had very low self-esteem and confidence, but that has grown over the years and I am finally comfortable in my own skin, happy with the person I have become. Let me tell you why.

When I was twenty-six and armed with a younger, more up to date specialist, he suggested trying IVF, with donor eggs from one of my sisters being my best option. As the youngest of five girls, I had a few choices but the next sister up from me offered to be my donor. She is not usually a huggy-feely kinda girl like I am, so when she said, 'I already have my son and don't want any more, and if there is one person that deserves to be a mum, it's you,' well I felt kind of special and I got all squishy and huggy, as she told me to get off her. I also had my long-time friend from high school offer to carry a baby for me as she had her three girls and wanted to help. As beautiful as that was, I declined, but I'm eternally grateful for her offer.

So, we started the process using my sister's eggs, and for those of you out there who have been through it, this needs no explanation. It is invasive, expensive and an emotional roller coaster, but a roller coaster that you jump on without hesitation if it means fulfilling that yearning void. Hell, I would have paid for that ride ten times over if it meant I would feel the warmth of a baby on my breast, that bond of a tiny human depending on me to give them the best life ever.

So, my next-up in age sister, bless her, got all the nasty injections. My husband got the joyous job of flipping one off in a tiny room with centrefolds all over the wall, putting it in a bag and ringing a bell for everyone to know he had just done his business! All I had to do was, I guess what most women do, lie there with my legs in the air ...oh and have a steel tube inserted in my hoo hoo.

Something that sticks in my mind to this day and makes me wonder what the outcome would have been years down the track, was when my sister's little boy asked a question. He said to her, 'So Mummy, if you give Aunty Lisa an egg and she grows it in her tummy, will it be my brother or sister or my cousin?' It did leave me with that thought of how do you explain to a child that 'you came from an egg from your aunty, you were made with daddy's sperm, but you grew in my tummy' - that was a whole new can of worms. Admittedly it did haunt me through the whole process that perhaps I was messing too much with nature? But I did it anyway ... haha.

Anyway, this rollercoaster ride went on for some years. In short, we collected sixteen viable eggs and had eight attempts at IVF. Of those, six of them worked, but failed within the first month of conception. It was heartbreaking, devastating and a total body slam. I comfort ate, maybe I comfort drank a bit too, and I cried myself to sleep on many occasions, for many years. Each time I would let the doctors pump me full of hormone injections, trying whatever we could to keep those little suckers in my inhospitable womb with my lemon lady bits, but they just wouldn't stick.

It's funny, the counsellors you see before you start this cycle tell you what to expect if you get pregnant, what to expect if it doesn't happen, but nobody told me what to expect if it worked then failed. I wasn't really prepared for that.

The first time I miscarried those precious little things, it was Day 28 after insemination. I woke up feeling a bit sick and rang all my sisters and they were excited because we all thought it was the start of morning sickness. I was so happy to feel sick. Then at lunchtime I ate a banana sandwich (you will see why this is important soon). About an hour later I got stomach cramps and went to the toilet and found I was bleeding. I freaked, like completely freaked and rang the fertility clinic. They told me not to panic, 'maybe it was the eggs settling in' as that happens sometimes, apparently. I should go home and rest. So I called a cab and hopped in. It was February and about thirty-eight degrees in the shade. The cab was stifling hot, I was sweating and crying and feeling like shit. About fourteen kilometres into the twenty kilometre, trip I felt like I was going to vomit. I said to the cabbie, 'Stop the car I'm going to vomit.' He looked at me with fear and I could see him counting the dollars if I did it in the cab! So he pulled over as soon as he could. I remember thinking, it was weird how with all that grass verge, he stopped across some poor bugger's driveway. I didn't have time to get the seatbelt off so I leaned on a weird angle out the door and vomited my small intestine up! All the deliciousness of that earlier banana sandwich was not quite the same when it hit the boiling pavement at fifty kilometres per hour. The smell that came back at me was what I imagine gorilla spew would smell like. To top it off, the weird angle I was leaning, along with my stomach convulsions lead to one thing- a giant fart, which would have blown directly into the lovely Indian cab drivers face. I was too ill to apologise but I did think at the time that this would be a funny story some day! In case you haven't guessed yet, I hide my pain with humour. It is the only way I can deal with things that hurt so much that I want to crawl into a hole and never come out.

At this point, can I add that everybody comes to comfort the female in these times, but forgets about the male and how he may be feeling. Contrary to popular belief, they do have feelings. I remember my husband putting on a brave face, holding me close while I cried my heart out, and when I asked how he was, he said, 'I'm fine, don't worry about me. I read the about the percentages of the chances of this working so knew it would be a longshot. But it's different for you because you carry the child.'

Later that night, after crying myself to sleep, I woke to a faint whimper in the night and realised it was my husband, quietly crying out his grief and loss when he thought I was sleeping. To this day, I'm not sure he knows I heard but I needed to let him grieve in his own way and give him the space I also needed to process. Never forget, the man is affected in the process just as much.

I worked in an IT department of a bank back then, in a predominately male environment, all of whom had children. So when I came back to work after the first failed IVF attempt, they were all unsure how to act. They avoided eye contact and emailed me instead of coming and having the usual witty banter every day. Generally they were so uncomfortable that I put my big girl's panties on, sucked it up and tried to joke around with them and tell them I was ok. I realised after doing this a few times that in my strange way of wanting to make everyone else happy and comfortable I was depriving myself of the need to grieve for my losses. After about try number four, I walked in, stood in front of them and said, 'I am struggling, I am upset, but I can't help it and I'm not sorry for being like this. Don't ignore me, please talk to me like you usually would, as it will help,'…and so they did. Why didn't I just say that in the first place?

One of the other defining moments for me during the whole process, was the day I miscarried attempt number five … on the same day my sister-in-law gave birth to a beautiful little boy. I cried happy and sad tears all at once. I have never missed seeing new family babies in hospital, so I braced myself and went in the next day to meet my new nephew. My sister in law was shocked to see me, and a little uncomfortable, but for me it was very cathartic. It is a blessing to have a baby, no matter what, and I have never felt the 'woe is me' when someone in my family had a child. My mind doesn't work like that because it's nobody else's fault I can't have a child, so they should not feel bad for celebrating their success. I admit, I did walk out of the hospital and have a cry in my car but I am so glad I did it and right there, in that moment, I realised I am stronger than I ever gave myself credit for. I was damn proud of myself and I'm not gonna lie about it. Sometimes it's not just about me, it's about the people around me and the people I love as well. A newborn baby is a time of celebration, no matter who they belong to.

So through all the sadness, the excitement and the whirlwind that it was, I'm glad we did it. Not to try is admitting defeat. It was an experience and it allowed us both to grow as humans, to appreciate the things we DO have in life and try not to dwell on what we couldn't have. I'm still excited to this day, twenty-five years later, when I hear of someone who has had a successful IVF birth and am happy to share my story with people considering it, encouraging them to give it a go. It may or may not work, but it's a shot isn't it?

Adoption or fostering were discussed between my husband and myself and thrust at us as suitable alternatives by well-meaning others, bless them, but it wasn't something my husband wanted to do. There were also a few people in our lives who didn't think it would be a good idea to adopt at 40 years of age, but I knew if I pushed hard enough, I could have forced him into it. I know if they put a tiny baby in his arms he would have loved it like nothing else on earth. But to force that situation on anybody is not right. While his reasons may not have made sense to me (although if I'm truthful I could see his point), I had to respect the decision. So that was the end of that.

Perhaps one of the most poignant things my husband said at the end of all this was that maybe we should stop looking to adopt or foster, and concentrate on all the kids in our family. Maybe our role in life is to provide a safe haven for them, a place for the kids to come for a break from their parents and for their parents to have a break from them. Maybe that's what we are supposed to do.

It was a light bulb moment for me. I had never thought of it this way and was surprised that he had, but he's always been the deep thinker in this relationship. I'm more the forgetful Dory who floats through life thinking of rainbows and lollipops. His take on this made me love him that tiny bit more because it took away some of the guilt I felt about depriving him of being a father, and make no mistake, he would have been a fucking good one!

As I write this story at fifty-two years and ten months of age, I am proud aunty to fourteen nieces and nephews and another four step nieces/nephews, thirteen great nieces and nephews (and at least one beautiful little soul who was too special to make it all the way to earth). I love them all and I would stand alongside their mums to protect those cubs any day.

I am also second mum to a lot of extended family and friend's kids. I would not change this for all the milk in a cow's udder! There is something overwhelmingly fulfilling when I can do things for the kids that perhaps would not have been possible if I had my own kids. I am so incredibly grateful for the mums and dads who have allowed me to be part of their kids' lives, who have allowed me to help shape them into the humans they have become.

I have come to terms with not being a biological mum. I have come to terms with the fact that I will never be a grandma. I have come to terms with the fact that I'm not perfect, and I'm okay with that.

There is an age old saying that people come into your life for a reason or a season. They come to share an experience or help you through an event, to teach you a life lesson. They may stay a day, a week, a year, or if you are lucky they stand by your side for life.

But each and every encounter and experience you have in life shapes you. It can make you falter, it can change your plans and it can make you stronger if you let it. I have had some life-altering times in my life. The IVF was the first. Then the death of my dad when I was twenty-seven; watching the man I looked up to fade away over three months to the big C. The death of my mum when I was fifty after she battled Alzheimer's for a couple of years; both of us crying when she realised the first time she couldn't remember my name. A marital hiccup when I was forty, (that's a story for another day…) and the process I went through to forgive the people involved and realise my own fault in this. Each of these were big events for me.

But for each of these events, there were people around me that had been there for a while. There were also some people who came into my life at those times. There were even some who I thought would be there, who left or whom I felt slightly let down by. I was held up by some and let down by others. I hold no grudges anymore (I may have for a bit, I wouldn't be human otherwise), but I also came to realise that whilst these events were the centre of my life, they were not the centre of everyone else's life. Everyone has their own things they are dealing with, and it was wrong of me to think that I should be their priority. How dare I? It made me question my own actions and whether I have always been the person I should or could have been. There are always two sides to everything.

During the IVF and other things in life, I learnt valuable lessons, and I walked away stronger EVERY TIME. My friendships became stronger, my beliefs became stronger, and the experience I could pass on to others to help them through similar situations became more realistic (rather than being based on my uneducated opinion). I realised I could harness my life experiences and use this to empower other women who have similar experiences, so they can find their 'shine' again.

So I guess the moral of my story is that when life throws you those lemons, add a large dash of vodka, a splash of soda, and drink the hell out of it! You only live once so make it count.

Be true to yourself, believe in yourself, and take every opportunity life throws at you. If that isn't good enough for everyone else, who cares?

My life is no worse and no better than anyone else's. We all have our different shit to deal with. It is neither less nor more important than anyone else's, but it's mine.

I have learnt a lot, had some curve balls thrown at me, but it's all part of my journey; it's made me who I am today. And I finally realised something along the way …

I am me, and that is enough. I AM woman, hear me roar!

I am a Rising Matriarch.

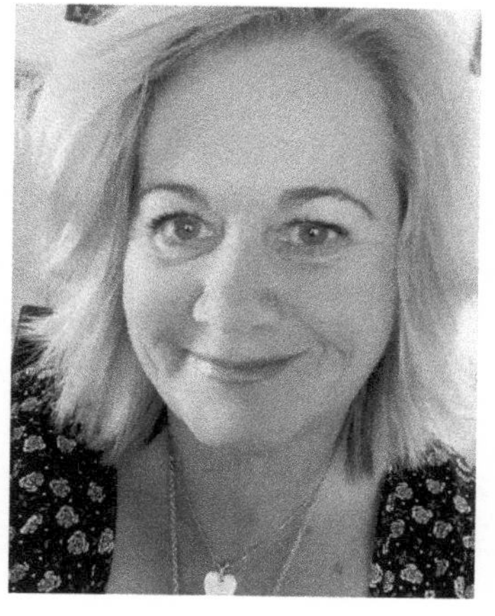

Lisa Johnson

Hiya, I'm Lisa and I'm thrilled to be part of this book and share one of my life stories with you. I was born one of five girls, obviously to a good catholic family! I grew up in a loving household with the usual sisterly love/hate things going on and was blessed with firm but loving parents with strong family values. That didn't stop me getting in a little bit of trouble as a teenager though, but when you grow up in a country town there isn't much to do, so trouble can find its way to you.

For some of my formative teenage years, my parents had an Ampol Roadhouse in Miami, south of Mandurah in Western Australia, home of "the Miami Monster" burger, which saw plenty of strapping young surfies come in every morning waiting for the breakfast of champions. It was here that I guess I developed of love of food and cooking, something that haunts my waistline a little everyday. I love to create - Food, poetry and writing- which is why this is an exciting venture for me.

That's not what I do for a living though. After years in the corporate rat race at a bank, then a law firm, I took leave of all that and headed into the humanity field. For the past 14 years I have worked with people with disabilities, helping them find and maintain satisfying employment. For me this is very challenging yet rewarding field. Their success is my success, and I get such a joy about being able to help change someone's life, by helping them achieve their goals. It's one of the best feelings in the world. My work, in some ways has been very cathartic for me as it allows me to use the love and energy a mother usually reserves for children in a positive way to help the community. Transference I believe they call it.

I am happily married, live in the burbs, and enjoy a healthy work-life balance. On weekends I paddle board and waterski and my husband and I have taught many of our family and friends to enjoy this fun watersport. I have a passion for AFL football and support my beloved Fremantle Dockers (opposing supporters will tell you that someone has to support them), and go to every game every season. We are yet to win a Grand Final but I'm hoping that before I go to heaven (or hell) it will happen. I also love shopping, for anything or for anyone. I love laughter and cracking jokes, it keeps me sane (or insane depending on who you listen to).

My purpose in this book is to help people realise that no matter what life throws at you, you can rise above it, learn from it, and use it as life experience to help others. I hope you enjoy it.

Love and light xxx

The Long Way Home

Michelle Duke

Have you ever found yourself in a downward spiral with a locked aim at what it is your soul desires? I found myself in a state of tunnel vision, unable to break away from the goal. I was robotic in nature, all the while my insides were aching for the one thing I could not bring to life. Multiple miscarriages had me struggling to keep my head above the surface of day-to-day life. I had disconnected from my body and felt my womb was more like a tomb, even though I had experienced the miracle of two successful pregnancies.

It was the repetitive failures following the birth of my second child that had me in a lock hold. I was fighting my body, willing it to follow through from conception, yet like clockwork I would begin to get the tell-tail signs around week ten. With each loss, another piece of me was gone too.

The desperation to bring to earth the little soul I knew was waiting on the other side, consumed me. I was a zombie to the rest of my life; routine kept me feeling safe and in a protective bubble that this was normal. Miscarriage will impact between 10-25% of clinically recognised pregnancies and while it is something that many women experience, it is often not talked about. You box it up and file it away in the 'Do Not Open' section of your memory bank.

On the topic of miscarriage, I would like to point out this is my own personal account with the impact it had on my relationships, that of my marriage, my children, friends, family and most importantly myself. I cannot speak for anyone else that these losses impacted, but what I can tell you is, to this day, it is a work in progress.

Unable to trust my intuitive ability any longer, I relied on the advice given to me by a psychic, who would blur the lines of her profession and claim friendship with me. I lost myself in this friendship believing this woman held the answers to my happiness. This dysfunctional relationship had me buying false hope, reading after reading. I laugh now at the perfect chaos that was brewing and how deliciously easy it was for her to instil fear into me. There were a few occasions that I would pay for her guidance and she would in turn reply that the reading was too bad to share with me; no refund, just a promise that when things changed in my situation, she would read for me again.

While I was focused on squaring things up with the Cosmos, I was ignoring the elephant in the room. My husband was withdrawing from our family more and more due to the living arrangements of his older children, and his inability to address his emotional upset. Hindsight is a wonderful thing, and looking back now, the Universe was really offering me a moment to pause and reflect on what was happening around me. Yet my opportunity to draw from this and see how his withdrawal was also a reflection of my own, was lost to me.

In true stubborn form, I pushed on, determined to get my prize no matter the cost. And if a price had to be paid, I surely did. My Guru upon hearing of my surprise pregnancy sent me grim news, if I were to stay, 'the baby would die.' Our household was wound so tightly from unexpressed feelings, tension, and exhaustion. As a habitual people-pleaser and domestic abuse survivor, my natural default setting was to keep the man happy at all cost. To be fair this man is kind, often gentle and would never raise his hand to me, yet my need to keep the peace meant that our communication was usually a one-and-a- half way street… I would share my thoughts and his opinion was final.

It had not always been this way. We started our relationship on equality; both sole parents with full-time custody of our children, both working through mediation with the other parent to our child, or children in my partner's case. We held an understanding that is not often found when you have children to bring into new partnerships. We worked hard to treat the children fairly. I felt this was the bond that would hold us together; something we would grow from no matter how much was thrown our way, and believe me it was thrown.

Sadly, not everyone who leaves a relationship is willing to let go completely of any perceived control they have over the other party. From the moment we began to date, interest from the ex was resumed in how the children were cared for and a more consistent visitation schedule took place. This was fantastic for the children who so desperately wanted to connect with their birth parent, and it gave us opportunity to get to know each other without all children on deck. The circumstances were different for my child however, with a combination of domestic violence, substance abuse and mental health issues, safety was of great concern.

The micro-management and dictatorship being attempted by the birth parent was a challenge. When faced with situations where you are being attacked for caring for another's children, it is hard to remain true to your core ethics. I struggled in high school with the politics and bitchy nature you often hear with groups of women, I even found completing an apprenticeship in a female dominant industry hard work. I do not understand the jealousy and need for gossip and I will do my best to remove myself from these situations as best I can; this has included saying good-bye to life-long friendships when my trust and character has been used against me.

If we all draw upon our core ethics, we will never find ourselves lost for what to do. It has been a life journey to understand what my values are. Truest to my heart is that of sisterhood; I will raise another woman up and *never* take opportunity to tear her down. So often I meet women with sisterhood wounding from this very issue. We have been played against each other for far too long and it is high time that we rise up and put an end to this petty squabbling amongst ourselves. We are being divided, distracted, and demoted in our power and authority, by this very issue.

Blending a family is never an easy path yet, if all adults maintained their focus on the children and continued to communicate openly with one another, the lives of our children would be better for it. We are, after all, role models for the future generations. It was always my intention that each child felt safe, heard, and loved by me and I know I did the best I could with the tools I had at the time.

As if I needed an extra push down the path of fear, my doctor had called me into his surgery for an important meeting while I was eighteen weeks along. My twelve-week scan had been misread and there was a chance of complications, I needed to do an amnio test that day, as I was too far along to wait. I had attended this appointment solo, so the decision fell to me directly and I refused, the risk of another loss far outweighed the possible outcomes from the testing. This was the first sign I was trusting myself again.

Each day I would connect with this little miracle in my belly and I knew they were perfect, just the way they were, I did not need the test to confirm this. What I did need was support from my partner for making this decision and allowing me the space to meet with all the degrees of emotions that rose, and to feel safe from the unknown. I asked, I was rejected. The tension in the house became increasingly painful and the words of this Guru echoed in my mind … Leave or your baby will die.

While his hand would never be raised to me, his rage was made known as he spate spiteful words at my son and one afternoon, even threatened a punch to the head. My son was twelve and was being called a liar due to previous deceit, bringing to a head the disharmony felt amongst us all. Safety was breached, a line crossed and when attempts to talk of the occurrence were still met with hostility, the words fell from my mouth, 'maybe we need a break.'

The next morning, he was gone, and the choice made for me.

In life you will find yourself back in a familiar situation time and again, a spiral cross-section. It is like the punchline to a joke you have not heard. So here I was again, single and pregnant, only this time I had two others to care for. Finding a place to live when you are expecting a child with the added tag of being a single mother is not the easiest. Thankfully, I had family that could help, so we moved closer to them and away from my husband.

Funny enough the friendship with this Guru fell away not long after the birth of our child. My husband was there for her arrival, purely by chance as it was Easter, and we had continued to maintain open lines of communication. Separation was not my desired outcome, but it was one that was needed for us to both look at what we wanted in life.

This space between us gave me a voice. I had been feeling stuck in a town that no longer filled me with joy. I had felt unjustly treated by his family along with his ex-partner, and he would not speak up on my behalf. I was far away from friends and family that could offer support. This was an opportunity to create change and I would not let it pass me by.

Prior to the birth of my first child, I had met a woman named Rainbow; a kinesiologist. 'What is that?' is the usual response to this modality. I had asked her that exact question, to which she suggested I try it out rather than her explain it. So, I tried it out and I absolutely loved our sessions. It was a modality that I felt I could do, yet I was just finishing up my hairdressing apprenticeship and expecting a child, oh and I was also doing that solo, so looking into kinesiology courses was not on my agenda that year.

Remember that spiral cross-section? Here I was, now with three children, I had decided I was not going back to hairdressing for many reasons, the main one being my hands and wrists would ache from full days of work and I felt I was not offering the level of change my clients would be truly seeking. I had spotted a kinesiology college was holding an open day and I decided to check it out. This turned into doing their mini weekend taster, followed by three years of study, finishing with an Advanced Diploma in Kinesiology.

There is a deep feeling of satisfaction for achieving something that you never thought would happen. It took me fourteen years and three children to return to that initial dream of studying this modality. I pushed through multiple hurdles, in those few years all the while investing in me.

I lost and found myself time and again, each layer of my identity was being stripped away in those lectures. I found that through studying kinesiology I was also healing myself from subconscious programs that had been playing out in my life. This was the nectar I needed to rebuild myself.

My husband and I had been living separated for nearly four years at this stage and I was once again over this half-life situation. Were we all in, or not? Something needed to change again, a whisper to the Universe was sent out. I called for a decision to be made. I was not returning to his hometown, there was no support, and I would be isolated once more from my friends and family.

As if he had caught my whisper, he announced one day that he was done with work, with living in that town and with being away from us all! Excited by his bold moves, I offered my support and eagerly awaited his response. Men seeking change do not respond well to excitement I must say… It was a glorious six weeks of looking at all the possibilities and where we could venture off to find our place in the world.

Survival of the species is deeply imbedded in our reptilian brain along with the desire to reproduce! The structure of how we do life and what the goal is varies from person to person.

My husband's decision to leave his job was a huge gamble, one that shocked even him. It was not a long-lived one and he returned to his employer. I often wonder what life would be like had he continued his forward action and taken the risk to leave that part of his life behind him. I was starting out as a small business at the time with my new modality, so financially, I was not as secure as he would like for this seemingly risky move.

A more consistent roster was put in place that would make us feel as though we were a family once more. As unwilling as I was to return to his hometown, I still yearned for a home that could provide space for us. Living in the suburbs had me feeling like a caged bird. You could hear the TV next door and smell them cooking meals. The patch of grass out the front was not safe enough for my young children to play, without the risk of them running onto the road or worse a car coming into the garden.

The more I deepened back into trusting myself, the louder my desire for a simple life became. Growing up I would visit my grandparents on their slice of heaven and enjoy time with my cousins. Often you would find us hiding in the mulberry tree making our way through the fruit and occasionally playing a game of mulberry tag. We would return to our Nan who would send us back to the tree to bring the unripened fruit back to clean ourselves, along with the clothes. Such fond memories of those times.

This was the lifestyle I wished for my own children and for the potential grandchildren to come. We had worked towards this dream some years before, purchasing just over five acres outside of the Toodyay townsite. We would take the kids there on weekends while we cleared the property ready for the coming summers. While it was limited to a shed, tank and a flushing toilet this was a place where dreams could grow.

In 2017 I set about calling in our new home. During the turbulent times dealing with the parent of my stepchildren, I remember my husband telling me she had warned him about me. 'She always gets what she wants,' were her words. I still laugh to this day about this warning because it is true. When I set my mind to something, I will ensure I reach that goal, and bringing us our new home was no different.

I remember finding a guided meditation that was designed to assist in attracting what you desired. It was to be done for seven days in a row and as I enjoy guided meditations, I felt this was easy enough to achieve. With nothing to lose and so much to gain I started. Each night I would listen and go through the processes instructed along the way. I was clear on my intent; we were to have the house and land at a price that was comfortable for us.

Day five into this meditation and I receive a frantic bunch of messages from my son. I had been uncontactable due to final assessments for my Advanced Diploma, so when I switched my phone back on, I was bombarded with missed calls and one-word text messages. Calling him back did not help much either, he was in shock.

Around 4pm that day in May, a BMW had managed to park itself into my front bedroom, creating a new water feature along with it. My son was the only one home at the time; a true blessing for he was in the back of the house, in his room, far away from any possible danger. He had thought the sound was another car hitting the letterbox of the house two doors down, something that had happened a little too regularly in the time we had lived on this road. Today however, it was our turn to be the subject of neighbourhood talk, with a prized BMW protruding from my window.

I arrived with my youngest two to find my home filled with cars and people. It was an overwhelming sight to behold. My son, still not yet calmed from his first-hand accounts, paced the road. My mum, who lived only ten minutes away, was there also. Had this been any other day the outcome could have been vastly different. Often my youngest would fall asleep around this time, while I would be starting dinner. I would place her onto my bed so the lounge was still free for the rest of us to use without waking her.

Chaos proceeds change and this event, while inconvenient was the change I was seeking. Puzzle pieces fell into place. Thirteen weeks of displacement from the BMW collision, until we moved into the house we would make our home. I never completed the rest of that guided meditation, but I knew whatever forces I had been working with at the time answered my call.

From this place we have begun to build dreams into reality. It has been a beautiful space to nurture our relationship, our family and ourselves. I have found the slowing down of life and again connecting into nature is what fills my soul the most. It is from this space I invite others to seek out their soul's desires. It may not be easy, but it will be worth it. If you can dream it, you can create it. No longer do I seek guidance outside of myself. If I do need a sounding board, my closest of friends, my soul sisters are the ones who I will speak with. Sisterhood is one of my most important connections outside of my family and it is these amazing women that continue to support my big dreams and crazy ideas, just as I do theirs. And this is what the world needs more of - soul sisters.

If at times you find it hard, hold my hand I will be here with you. If at times you struggle to believe in yourself, hold my hand, I believe in you. And if at times you forget who you are, turn to me so I can reflect back to you who you are.

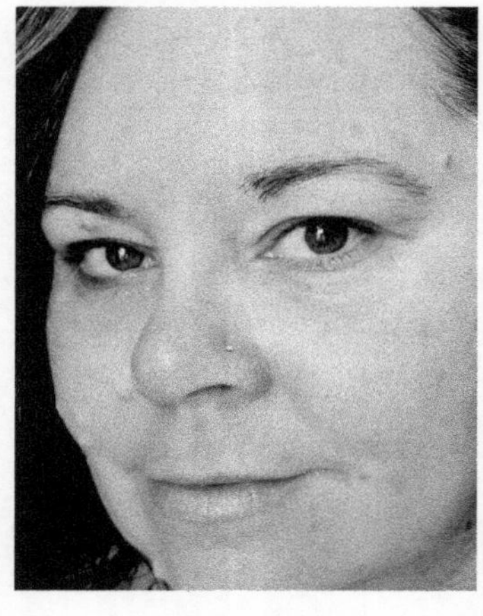

Michelle Duke

I have long been a seeker of Universal truth. I embraced this craving to understand on a deeper level the Universe for myself which has found me walking the path of the Mystic, Healer and Alchemist more deeply. I am a dedicated Priestess to the New Paradigm of consciousness evolution; this has seen me study multiple styles of Energy Medicine, holding an Advanced Diploma in Kinesiology as well as being an Intuitive Intelligence Trainer and Teacher.

Born in the coastal city of Bunbury, Western Australia when it was still a sleepy town, I spent many summer holidays returning there and have fond memories of my nan and pop's house where all the cousins would spend hours in the mulberry tree, being wild and free. While being baptised Church of England long before I could choose my own path, as a family we did not attend church often. Nature has always been my religion. Following the seasons along with the ebb and flow of the moon has been my anchor into the physical world.

Guilty of spending far too long outside of day-to-day life I have always been a day dreamer, shooting star wisher and if I could ever find the end of that rainbow, I will let you know what is on the other side! My school report cards were constantly noting of my ability to succeed if only I could focus on the task at hand. It is a testament that focus comes when it is something that makes your heart sing.

Sharing life moments with others is natural to me, I feel we best learn from each other. While I prefer the art of story telling verbally, I feel there is something majickal about sharing via the written word.

www.michelleduke.com
Instagram: @michelleduke.intuitivealchemy
Facebook: IntutiveAlchemist

No Wrong Turns

The Road to Freedom

Nellie Barnett

When I proudly declared at the dinner table one night that I had committed to co-authoring a book, my daughter's face lit up with unprecedented delight. I shouldn't have been surprised, really – we are a TV free family, so Sophia's (or Byx as she has recently re-named herself) most favourite chill zone is books. As in, she DEVOURS them by the minute and has nearly out-read the library and local book stores. She also writes her own stories, on the vintage baby-blue typewriter we found her for her tenth birthday (she'd been asking for one for years.) 'Can I help?!' came her immediate exclamation, it wasn't really a question. And so, knowing the innate wisdom I have witnessed flow from the mouths of babes over the years, my answer – Yes. I have included some of her contributions in this chapter. I hope they bring you as much simple goodness, insight and teachings as she has brought to me.

***

If you've ever had a tears-of-joy orgasm, that was the feeling in the moment when it hit me – it was like every force of nature you can imagine, rolled up into one all-consuming, deliciously cleansing, tidal wave of relief and realisation.

I had been spending 90% of my time and energy on the wrong people.

BYX SAYS: If you feel sad around someone, you can still love them, but don't need to spend your time and energy on them.

Not that they were 'wrong' by birthright, but they were most definitely wrong for me, and I for them.

The memory of the moment is still so vividly clear. Like that tidal wave was making love to a lightning bolt at the time it struck me, it imprinted into all levels of my consciousness and exploded little baby balls of liquid electricity into every cellular particle of my being.

I was literally in the middle of no-where when it happened. Somewhere in the red desert-y goodness near the South Australian & Northern Territory border, where ironically, my two year-old daughter, our 1970s caravan and I, were about ninety degrees and fifteen hundred kilometres off track from where we had originally planned to be.

You could say, I basically took the best wrong-turn of my life when, for whatever reason, at the last split second, I 'failed' to turn left at the major Port Augusta intersection toward the Nullarbor & Western Australia (as I had already marked out on my maps). Instead, I went straight up and onto the Stuart Highway towards the Northern Territory. Call it my Divine Sliding Doors moment.

BYX SAYS: Can we do it again??!

That 'wrong' turn, and the following tidal-wave-lightening-orgy moment, marks a distinct before-and-after line in the book of my life.

If you were to hear my 'before' story, the one from the mouth of my victim state, it might sound something like this ...

Born into an out-of-wedlock and less than ideal situation, I perceived from a young age that I wasn't meant to be here, and I was unwanted, right from conception.

My first sexual encounter was then experienced somewhere around the age of six. To be completely honest, I don't even know what to call it. Rape doesn't quite seem to fit, but at six, in a room with four males of varying ages, it certainly wasn't consciously consensual, or legal either.

The truly horrific part of that piece of my story is not the event itself, but the feelings that overwhelmed me on the walk home. I was evil, dirty, broken, so very, very naughty and if my Mum & (Step) Dad ever found out, I was surely going to be dis-owned, kicked out of home, sent off for adoption and no one was ever, ever, ever going to be able to love me from that point forward.

We'd been going to Church every Sunday since I was two years-old, and I knew this was about as bad a sin as one could commit. I was damaged goods and going to hell. In the meantime, I saw myself as deemed to live out hell on earth, in my own mind, as punishment.

Coincidentally, my younger sister was also born around this time, so effectively, as I saw it then, I had already been replaced by someone pure and untarnished anyway. I would not be missed. A disgusting, disobedient child like me, who was unwanted from the beginning, had no place in this world.

The impact of this event on my psyche would be unconsciously active, and as a result, play out in the reality I created every day for the next twenty-four years.

It showed up in every facet of my life.

My early teens saw me experience several cases of inappropriate conduct and molestation by older male family 'friends,' which left my head spinning and further cemented my beliefs around being a dirty, damaged, evil piece of work.

Everywhere I went, I felt like a misfit. And because I believed that, school proved tough too. I was bullied and taunted often, even more so, because I genuinely enjoyed learning and worked hard. Looking back, my perfectionist tendencies were likely a ploy for attention, and validation from those in 'higher positions;' an attempt to gain the approval of my parents and teachers. Perhaps if I worked hard enough and got good enough results, my soul could be redeemed and I wouldn't be disowned after all. Perhaps my existence would be validated if I was 'successful.'

My first adult relationship, at seventeen, with a twenty-eight year-old, was a two-and-a-half year emotional roller coaster ride that involved mental, physical, sexual, financial and drug abuse. I stayed, addicted to the drama and circumstances because I truly believed at the time that I was not worth any better; 'this was probably just how relationships were meant to be,' for me, anyway.

By the time that relationship finally ended properly, I had left home and built my identity and life around his, and he stripped me of the lot of it; our car, cat, home, friends.

I had been naive enough to shift my entire life into his name, and so it went. I took the BBQ I'd bought him one day, just as a 'something,' and he threatened me with violence and legal action. I was too exhausted to fight, so I returned it and walked away with nothing.

And then came the self-abuse.

At nineteen, with very little family support, I simply didn't understand the pain I was feeling. For the life of me, I couldn't make sense of being able to FEEL a pain, but not SEE it. So I set about making sense of it, making it visible. I tried my hand at cutting – it didn't really cut it for me though (#pardonthepun). Tearing my skin open with my own fingernails brought some satisfaction, but it was in smashing my head against the wall until it was like a bowl of fruit-pulp and slapping myself in the face 'til it burned red and raw, where I found relief. Now, I had a good reason to cry, one that made sense from an external perspective. A pain I could see, and yet, ironically, would continue to hide from the world.

Somehow, I made it through that phase alive. Probably mostly in thanks to ecstasy, dancing and a new group of people in my life.

I was also lucky enough, to have an innate, underlying sense of trust in some sort of bigger picture and plan, an inkling of the vast universe and infinite power that lay deep within me. A taste, on the tip of my tongue, that there was something better, that a happier life was possible.

BYX SAYS: There IS a land out there, that we can't see, but that does always have a happy ending, and where all Spirits are good.

So I read some books, did some courses, explored some philosophies, and things started to shift a little. The jewels and hope of a life less traumatic and more beautiful began to appear in my field of vision, as I began to create the neural pathways required to see them.

But still, the old patterns persisted.

Cycles of badly-chosen sexual encounters, low self-value, never being satisfied in my job, rocky friendships. You, know, the usual blah, blah, blah.

I fell in love, like, properly in love, once, amongst it all.

Then I left, to go travel the world for a year.

I thought we would stay together somehow and it would all work out when I got back.

Which it didn't.

Took me fifteen years to get over that one.

Oops. Naïve much? Ouch.

Started my own business, a restaurant, at the age of twenty-two.

Fell pregnant with Sophia at twenty-six, whilst trying to tick 'one night stand' off of my bucket list. (Failed bucket list attempt).

Sold the restaurant when Sophia was eight months old, at a huge financial loss.

Nearly went bankrupt.

In and out of, an again, very unhealthy relationship with Sophia's father, which came to completion when she was about eighteen months old.

Got deeply entrenched in the sports skydiving world which was a fascinating, adrenalin-based, uniquely-charactered space, filled with equal amounts of joy & toxicity / open-mindedness & judgement. A giant candy jar of every sort of sweet and sour surprise you can imagine.

Made some mistakes there, which I feel were very harshly judged, even when others involved in the team-effort-mess walked free. The term 'scape-goat' comes to mind.

Spent the next six months exhausting myself with trying to 'get back in with the crowd,' tearing myself apart again with all the 'why am I not good enough?' lines.

Until the day I went 'Fuck this.' jumped in my vintage caravan with a two year-old Sophia, hit the road, and didn't turn left.

FREEDOM.

What you've just read is the sob story, the 'poor me,' the victim story, and there's more to it – a lot more. But to be honest, it kind of bores me to write about it from that perspective now.

It was certainly real (and definitely not boring) at the time, every moment of it, all the pain, all the grief – all completely valid, just as yours is.

But I see it all so differently today.

Guess where I am at this time?

And more importantly, guess what is also accessible to you and every other divine being on this earth, at whatever precise movement one would come to choose it?

Joy.

Pure, fucking, tidal-wave-lightening-orgy, tearful-orgasm, standing-on-the-edge-of-a-cliff, internally created Joy.

FREEDOM.

BYX SAYS: Always look to your heart and the wisdom that is inside you.

Don't get me wrong – I don't shit rainbows and burp unicorns.

I still fuck up. Life hurts sometimes and I still cry, though those tears tend to be more joy than grief these days. And I'm not kidding myself, it's possible life might bring some unexpected hiccups yet and I may be tested on what I have created – touch wood, so far that's not the case.

But joy and happiness are my predominant internal state.

EVEN when the shit hits the fan and I'm a curled up mess of ugly tears.

The difference?

I know my story. I acknowledge my story. To write it now and read it over still elicits an emotional response. The pain was real, the pain was valid. The behaviour displayed by others involved was not and never will be OK.

But it doesn't MEAN anything to me anymore. It doesn't mean anything ABOUT ME.

I'm able to see a balance between the pain experienced, but also the benefits, value, learning and growth I was gifted through those same experiences. I see the divine order and timing in them, towards my personal evolution and the creation of the state of ecstatic, internal joy I now know is available to me at any moment. It's all there, in your experience too – you just have to choose to start seeing it.

FREEDOM

It was one of my first tattoos.

But I never realised until just lately, what a huge role in my life this word would play.

There had been moments, glimmers of it throughout the years, but it was really the move to leave Adelaide in the caravan (broke and with a two year-old on my own!), the split-second decision at that Port Augusta turn-off, and the desert-road realisation that, like I said, were the 'before and after' line in the sand of my life.

From there I embarked on not only a physical journey of almost twelve months on the road, completely free, but also a huge mental and emotional shift started to happen, and things really started to change.

I met my partner of now seven years, to whom I'm currently engaged and pregnant with! And while I may not burp unicorns, apparently, I am to marry and bear children to one. Seriously, you couldn't dream this guy up, though it seems that somewhere along the line, I did.

BYX SAYS: My heart bursts when I look Dad in the eyes, my family is the centre of my life.

I found 'home' as soon as Sophia and I hit the South West of WA in the caravan. And although we took a slight detour through Sydney for a few years, the region called me back so strongly that we purchased our first home here in 2016. Every step I take on the land around here feels like I've walked these paths a million times before. It's like the dirt, the trees and the ocean know me, remember me and welcome me, and I, them. It's not just the space here either. The people, the community we've called in and created, they get me. They love me for ALL that I am. No need to hide, fear or shame any part of myself anymore.

And after having moved through several businesses and careers, my soul purpose and passion began to become clear too.

The path I was choosing and the journey I was on, led me step-by-step right to the door (literally) of being introduced to something called German New Medicine, or Germanic Healing Knowledge.

Enter: The next pivotal part of my personal growth and evolution.

If you're into becoming the best, happiest, healthiest, joy-filled, internally sovereign and medically/system-free version of you that is possible, and you haven't heard of GNM / GHK yet, you're going to want to take note of this next part.

What is GNM / GHK?

Well, in short, it is a completely different way of understanding the psyche, brain, body, biology, dis-ease and wellness. GNM / GHK enables the individual to comprehensively understand the root cause of, and resolve their own symptoms, naturally, and in most circumstances, without ANY external influence (supplements, meds, other practitioners etc.)

It is the most empowering, independent and sustainable form of true healthcare and medical FREEDOM I have ever come across.

And it's what I now teach, work with and live by.

The principles of GNM / GHK (the "5 Biological Laws of Nature") show us that dis-ease, symptoms and illness are not some random break-down or mis-hap in the body, caused by some ferocious germ/microbe that is caught, or any other dis-empowering, external force. Neither are they faulty genetic hand-me-downs thanks to our parents. Rather, every physical and mental discomfort that shows up in the body, (bar accidents and poisoning) is the direct result of a specific moment in time; one where we experience something that we perceive to be a shock, a trauma, or catches us off guard. Not only that, but each of these physical or mental symptoms, each tissue adaptation, has a very distinct pattern AND a **specific** and **meaningful** biological purpose. They are all initiated in order to ASSIST the individual in times of unexpected distress. What does this mean for us?

It means > Fear of dis-ease and germs be gone!

It means > We can resolve our own symptoms by resolving the original distressing event, either in real-time or by changing our perception of the event.

It means> We can AVOID dis-ease and illness all together, just by being aware of our experiences and consciously choosing the way we see them.

But what the knowledge of GNM / GHK also gifts us, goes well beyond relief of and future-proofing ourselves against physical & mental dis-ease and symptoms.

It also gives us an exact roadmap of where we still need to resolve conflict, where we still need to work and heal, emotionally, in order to be our truest, most fulfilled, free and joyous selves.

Think Louise Hay's metaphysical theories, on DMT, with scientific backing and a solid basis in true biology and embryology. You'll be somewhere in the ball-park of the mind-blow factor of what I'm talking about if you imagine yourself there.

We are not separate to nature, we are part of it, and to witness this biological paradigm with a new understanding is to witness nature at work in the full extent of all her glory and power, holding us with loving intent.

This is where I truly began to remember my truth and power.

I AM nature at work, experiencing and loving herself.

I am an energetic particle of consciousness having a natural experience in a

Human container.

I am | You are | WE are.

How could something that profound and divine possibly be broken, dirty, damaged or faulty in it's very essence?

We are not born like that. Not even our experiences make us like that. But our PERCEPTION of those experiences, the meaning we attach to them, can make it SEEM like that.

Conditioning can make it seem like that. Lies, manipulation, ill-intentioned systems, media and organisations who stand to gain by holding a population in a state of disempowerment, external reliance, fear and absolution of self-responsibility, can make it seem like that.

The opposite of FREEDOM.

I urge you - denounce anything that makes you feel like this.

It's the ultimate form of terrorism.

Repel it, repulse it, boycott it, revolt against it with every cell of your being.

Move ONLY towards things that sound / smell / look / taste / feel like Freedom. It's there that you will remember the full extent of ***your*** truth and power.

BYX SAYS: We have a voice and we can use it. No one can rule us. We are our own adventure. Our Spirit can speak, it can shout, it can blaze.

I remembered my ***truth*** when I stopped trying to fit into places I was never meant to be. When I realised I was spending 90% of my energy on the wrong people. When I realised what it felt like to no longer care so much what other people thought of me. When I came to understand that other's perceptions of me are based on their own fear and pain. When I remembered what freedom tasted like. When I remembered I WAS nature herself.

I remembered my ***power*** when I realised that the only meaning something has, is the one we choose to give it – and that we can change that meaning at any given moment.

Nothing has ANY meaning, if we allow it to be so.

When I learned that my body and mind were not broken or faulty by design or by experience, but that she acts purely in accordance with what she knows, to help me survive. And that when she and I could assist each other out of survival mode, we could instead begin to THRIVE.

And the best punch line of all?

It's entirely possible that I don't know shit.

That every word I've shared here is wrong.

That I could do a full 180 and change, completely, tomorrow, or in the next minute even.

And so could you.

But isn't that such a beautiful thing?

And because of that …

I invite you NOT to believe a single word I say …

But to take what resonates, the parts that make your soul go 'Fuck Yes' - or even the parts that make you go 'WTF?!' Take whatever parts ***stir*** you, and go explore them for yourself. Try them on for size, see what fits and what works for YOU.

FREEDOM.

No mandates, no judgement of self or others, no one-size-fits-all.

Just keep an open mind.

And above all else,

Seek and embrace Joy, always.

Wishing you the ultimate state of health & happiness,

Nellie. Xx

BYX SAYS: This evening when I looked at the sky there was a golden haze on one side, with blue on the opposite and it made me feel free, and a joy swept over me.

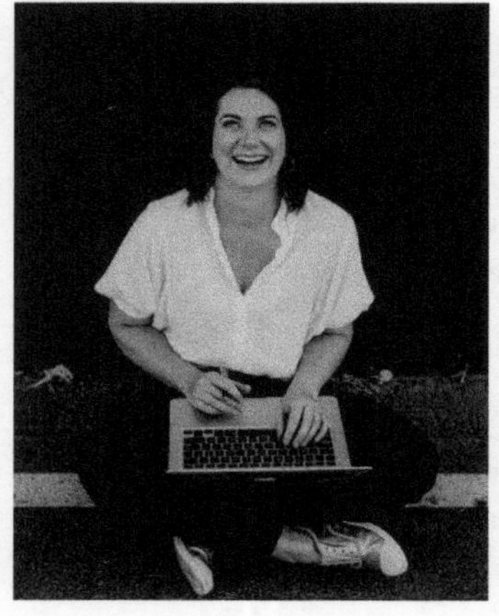

Nellie Barnett

Hey I'm Nellie!

Walking contradiction, in all the most fun ways. Lover of the vast array of emotions and adventures that the full spectrum of Human possibility and experience has to offer – and plenty that are seemingly outside of the Human realm too.☺

Mum to one Earth-side champion and another currently baking, I finally found 'home' five years ago with my Best Mates (Daughter and Partner) in the South West of WA, nestled among the bush, sea and vines of this beautiful land. After leaving my hometown in the Adelaide Hills in a caravan back in 2012, and embarking on the journey of a lifetime with my then two year old, the area 'called us in'.

I have always had a profound love of learning and Entrepreneurship and the two combined landed me with multiple certifications in the realms of mental and physical health and several of my own businesses ranging from flower sales on the sidewalk at age five, three cafes and other, side ventures along the way.

The evolution of my own personal development, studies and love for self-employment wove together to result in the manifestation of my soul-business, Nellie B Well established in 2016.

It is now my absolute joy to assist others to find health and happiness via sustainable, independent and natural means in my flagship offering: The New Earth Wellness Empowered Health Academy.

I believe very strongly in freedom of choice and speech, particularly when it comes to the medical world and am currently dedicated to educating freedom-seeking Humans in the application of Germanic Healing Knowledge (GNM), so they can create their own state of Wellbeing, without having to rely on external resources or the 'system.'

Alongside this, I also believe that life is to be lived, enjoyed, celebrated and that above all, we should seek joy and adventure in every moment possible. So, when I'm not teaching in the Academy and interacting with my students, you'll find me dancing like a dork in the kitchen with my family, tending to our co-op biodynamic farm garden, seeking out the lushest Champagne to sip on, exploring this world's fascinating plant-medicine specimens, gawking at an octopus for an awkward amount of time through a snorkel mask, getting messy playing with clay, baking something that calls for fresh double cream to enjoy with, or of course, with my nose in a good book.

I reject the title 'Healer' (no one can do that for you, other than you), and even teacher doesn't quite feel right to me.

What I am proud and delighted to offer you, is the opportunity to be guided back towards remembering what you already know to be true, before all the conditioning and 'stuff' happened. That is, the innate power, strength, beauty, divine nature and empowerment that lies right within you. I help you facilitate your own 'un-becoming' so can truly just BE. FREE.

Loving you for all that you are.

Nellie B. Xx

www.nelliebwell.com
www.wellnessacademy.nelliebwell.com
Instagram: @nelliebwell
Facebook: nelliebwell

The Power in You

Ninielia Marie

Who would have thought the one thing humans desire most in life is love, without realising that is the one thing we can provide to ourselves?

There is great sorrow and enormous pain etched in my soul, as I sit legs curled up, cradling them whilst rolling myself in a ball of mess. My scream comes from the pit of my stomach and echoes, sending vibrations trembling through my wearied body. Tears trickle down my face and then turn to a steady stream that could fill an ocean. I am tired beyond the desire for sleep, and as the exhaustion sets in, a sense of engulfing numbness overcomes the entirety of my being, although I can still feel the harshness of the cold floor beneath me. I watch the light through the window as the shades turn darker and day turns to dusk.

Hours have passed, as I look in the mirror and do not know the reflection looking back at me. It is as if there are two of me, one of which I do not want to hold onto, so I attempt to force this overwhelming sorrow out of me as I desperately search for a sense of peace within my raging soul. My eyes are as red as the deepest rose you could ever find, and my nose is so stuffy and blocked that I can hardly breath. I gasp for air in between my screams, as I drown in my own sorrow. The crushing sensation in my heart is sending shock waves through my body and I can anxiously feel the fire burning inside of me, as it surfaces inch by inch like a powerful storm in a midnight sky. The fiery lump gets so enflamed that it remains stuck in my throat creating a deep burning sensation that chokes me. I let out a soul-wrenching scream again, in attempt to set the roaring storm free.

I have been in this place many times before; where there are no lower depths of despair and even the deepest ocean does not compare to how unfathomable my sorrow is in these moments. I am lost and even in a vast and vibrant universe I feel alone and isolated in my misery. I feel as if I cannot go on. I want to go to a place I do not know of, where I can gain serenity. I scream out, 'I want to go…help me…. please help me…I want to go,' whilst uncontrollably sobbing and tirelessly searching for answers. In this moment I am completely and utterly depleted. The shame of how I feel in this moment triggers anger and guilt that reach beyond the depths of my control, so much so that I start to punch myself in the face as the energetic rage surfaces again. The impact leaves red markings on my already puffy face with swollen lifeless eyes staring back at me in the mirror again. The physical pain caused by my own fists to my face, does not compare to the pain in my heart and soul. I fear myself because I have no value for my face, nor for my heart, or even for my life. Who are you I wonder?

I turn the bathroom light off and take comfort in the solitude of the pitch-dark blackness of the night. My spirit is lost, and I struggle without fully understanding why. I search further and deeper for answers as my body gives in through fatigue and finally, I can think for a moment. I call out to my grandmother who has passed into the spirit world and she comes to me almost immediately. I am still rolled-up, but this time I feel a warm embrace, as if a soft rug has been placed over my tired body. She is comforting me. I finally fall asleep and she comes to me in my dream to remind me of my power. The power she has passed to me.

'What power?' you ask. The power to know that sometimes, the outer world will impact you so harshly that you forget who you are, you question your worthiness, and you revel in unloving sentiments towards yourself because of the judgement of others. 'What outer world impacts?' you ask: the one that requires you to be something you are not, and sets expectations that you must live up to the standards of a modern world and its patriarchal perspectives. One where society embraces masculinity over everything, as if every human to have ever walked this earth was not born of a woman in her most ultimate feminine power! The one that forces you to lose out on your own femininity, your power, dreams and identity.

'How do you get your power back?' you ask: through acceptance and compassion, for yourself and your circumstances. There is already too much judgement passed on through this world by others who are probably even more confined by the imprisonment of their negative thoughts, self-doubt, and lack of self-love. Do not fear the perspectives of others. Sadly, we know that society is ruled by perceived perfection over genuine authenticity. Void those benchmarks from your mind and heart. No more!! No more should you allow anyone to cast judgement over you and expect that you wear it like a badge of honour. The real pool of misfortune lies in a soul that is not who they choose to be, whilst standing sheepishly in someone else's shadows.

"So, was that the issue?" you ask. Was I wearing labels, branded on me by others? Did I validate my entire existence based on whether others thought I was loveable and worthy? Was I setting expectations on myself to please others? Was I allowing myself to only be influenced by those who were carrying their own traumas and not able to stand in their truth? Was I unequipped with the knowledge and ability to deal with my own past traumas? Was I struggling to heal? Yes. Did I need to learn to love myself? YES!!

The morning sun greets me through the slightly opened window-blind, and in the subconscious moments before I fully awake to the sounds of the birds chirping outside, I am dazed by the internal awareness of surreal peace that I welcome with all my heart. The light from outside that is glimmering through with radiance and warmth seems so bright due to my memory of the darkness of the past night. I thank my grandmother for comforting me. She is in the spirit world again, but her consciousness is universal, enabling her to travel through the realm of the spirit world to me transpiring light through the energies and frequencies of the cosmic universe. She will be connected to my spirit forever.

Slowly but surely, I recount the events of the day and night before and whilst sadness starts to emerge in a corrosive attempt to strangle me again, I stop it in its tracks, humbly knowing that I have made another day. There is something magical in the sense of coming out the other end alive. It is something to be truly proud of. Even the strongest of us have experienced overwhelming grief and sadness and no doubt questioned, even for a moment, if we have the strength to go on. There is no shame in that. In fact, there is enormous power, deep resilience, and phenomenal strength that comes through that journey. It reflects that you understand defeat and being helpless, but you still can find the courage to rise above the darkness into the light.

You need to trust in the universe and know, whilst in challenging moments you may not be able to control what is going on around you or within you, however you are still able to take comfort in knowing that with time, it will pass. Time will go on and change is inevitable. The sun will set and rise again, the stars will shine bright, the trees will shed their leaves, the monsoonal rains will come to cleanse the earth, and the seasons will flow on around you and through you. No one moment lasts forever, so lean into those challenging moments and give yourself the compassion and time you deserve. Be brave in the hope for a new day and graciously flourish in the opportunities it can provide because the potential is truly endless.

I clearly remember the days after the storm when I learnt to take everything in my stride. I began to heal through the hurt, and the pain led to power.

However, the process to gaining strength is undeniably not an easy process. Becoming strong is when you get knocked down and can get back up again. Those who are the strongest, become that way because they have more experience in rising after falling. They know the true essence of joy, because they have felt pain unbeknownst to others. You must realise that pain serves a purpose and that purpose, if you allow it, will create internal expansion like rays of sunlight. It will enable growth like bright rainbow streams with no end in sight. It will create transformative change, like the caterpillar into the beautiful butterfly about to give flight.

That morning as I lay in bed, I developed an acceptance that people will see me through their own lens. I learnt to understand that their perspectives have been informed by their journey, therefore it was unfair of me to internalise the views of others, because it represented who *they* were, not who I was, or who I chose to be.

I ask you to ponder for a moment.

Do you think those that cast judgment are compassionate?

Do you think those that display narcissistic behaviours do so out of genuine care and love?

Do you think those that do not know how to show love have love for themselves?

Do you think those that are bitter and angry care enough to grow into their own light?

Sadly, the answer is No. It is in this realisation I knew I had to be a constant reminder to myself, of everything that was beautiful and perfect about me, despite those who walked away when I needed them most. I began to realise that the real honour in life was in finding the courage to stand proudly in my own truth, power, and uniqueness.

So, I woke and made it out the other end, and now you ask, 'And then what?' I began to accept the ebb and flow, fall and grow, philosophy of life. I knew that my drive to discover 'who I am?' was not a stagnant destination I could ever simply arrive at and finally be healed. I knew that being true to myself was honouring the process, as much as it was about honouring myself, and the desire for an end outcome. I began to realise the best way to succeed in life, was to continuously accept my evolution with humbling grace.

But first I had to transition. I had to move. I had to let go of where I had been before and sadly, I had to understand there were people around me who triggered my emotional grief and influenced me in a way I did not want to be influenced anymore. I had to let go of those people, not because I did not love them, but because I knew they had been on their own journey, which clearly reflected where they were in their lives, and what their priorities were at the time. I was not a priority. I was criticised and never felt good enough, giving birth to self-doubt and subsequently striving to be more and do more, in search of acceptance and love. This was triggering me negatively, creating the fear and a belief I was not capable of receiving unconditional love. The triggers grew to bitterness and hate but I soon realised you cannot force people to love you in the way you desire, and as the saying goes, you can't fight fire with fire. I had to cut the cord between myself and others, with loving intent. I knew I had to embark on my own journey and they would take their own path too. This process of letting go was the hardest thing to deal with, and I grieved the loss of them for a long time as if they had died. The experienced sadness was profound because I still wanted to believe they loved me in their own way, but I also knew they were still learning to love themselves, and as such, they did not know how to show love in the way I needed it, without doubt, strain, or compromise.

'How does your environment, and the people in it, affect your life? you ask. I cannot stress enough how much those within your life and your surroundings will impact your ability to thrive or not. Sadly, people can love you, but not want what is best for you. Some people selfishly don't want you to grow. They fear change because they want you to be what *they* need you to be, and not what you want to be. They may even hate you for abandoning them, and become envious you are happy without them, whilst they still live in their denied misery. You must let go anyway. If you accept a place in someone else's book, you will never grow beautifully into the magnificent garden of your authentic self. Instead you will grow destructive weeds of anger, resentment, and hate towards them and yourself. Yes, growth is hard, but sitting in your misery in order to serve others is way harder. When you begin to discover your truth and light, a lot of people will not accept it. Again, societal norms consider intuition and emotional truth-telling as trouble-making. To that I say stay grounded in your soulful intuition and honour your truth, even if others don't accept it. Even if it means you must stand alone. Silence is the greatest killer of all, and if you silence your soul to please others, what worth is it to have one at all?

'What if you can't let go?' you ask. Sometimes the process of letting go takes time, a long time. You can't just wake up in the morning and let go of every person that has ever misjudged or mistreated you, or who is holding you back from fulfilling your own life's purpose or desire for love. What you can do is develop honouring boundaries. 'What are honouring boundaries?' you ask. It is drawing a protective line in the sand. The side you are on is your safe space with a clearly defined set of conditions allowing you to determine who, when and why you let people into your honouring space. You can stand firmly and confidently in what you will and will not accept from others, with the purposeful intent to protect yourself and your journey. Letting go a little at a time, is not failing this process. You will find as you loosen your grip on the situation, relief will come slowly but surely, making it easier to let go even further, until there is nothing left to hold on to.

I found it difficult to set boundaries at first. Most of the time I would feel bad because I believed it was selfish and the last thing I wanted to be was selfish, because I knew the impact of being around people who were. So instead, I learnt to understand, through trial and error and many failed attempts, you can be selfish in two ways; 1) in order to gain and 2) in order to give. My positive intent was the latter. I needed to be selfish in setting boundaries so I was able to protect myself like a fierce warrior goddess turned queen. I knew by doing so I could also protect, care and nurture those loved ones around me. I also learnt to set boundaries with loving acknowledgment and acceptance of who other people are and where you can best leverage off each other without unrealistic expectations or uncaring conditions.

'So how has this loving acceptance, process of letting go and boundary setting transpired in my life?' you ask. It has resulted in my own evolution and my awakening to a new dawn of possibilities. I have emerged into the light of my true self, whilst igniting greater levels of frequency, power and magnetic energy, enabling manifestation of everything that my heart truly desires. I can also tell you that my circle is small. I keep it this way because I have learnt that the greatest level of love I can gain is from myself, no one else. Over the years, my reliance on others has become less and I have surrendered any meaningless connections. My longing for acceptance by others is non-existent. My desire to gain a sense of security from others has miraculously vanished. I therefore encourage you to be mindful of who you let into your intimate space and your circle of love. My network though is broad, providing opportunity to gain knowledge, inspiration, wisdom, and motivation from others as and when I require it. I control this network, and the flowing tide of incoming and outgoing people, with acknowledgement that the universe will support this process in line with my desires and aspirations. Call it manifestation, fate or synchronicity. I trust that what is meant for me will be and I too will be called into people's lives as they need me.

Another thing I have found interesting and somewhat motivating is that you would be amazed how many people admire your authenticity, secretly or not. I have had many people message me over the years saying how I have influenced them, how they admire my confidence and courage, how I positively contributed to their lives, and provided much needed motivation at times of despair. For some of those people, I literally didn't have the slightest idea I had that level of impact in their lives. 'So what?' you ask. Well, you see, honouring your truth enables and empowers others to do the same. I am an ordinary woman with many things to be grateful for. I have many achievements in my life but have also gone through heartache and pain. It goes without saying that my biggest achievement has been the discovery of my power and I am heartened that others are enriched by my presence, and as a result, my influence.

Today, I stand proud and tall in who I am, flaws and all. I am unapologetically me. I have developed clarity in who I am, consistency in my approach to loving myself, and a commitment to showing others the way to their truth and light. I am sincerely grateful for the journey I have been on, particularly those nights on my bathroom floor, which led me to be grounded in my truth. It's strange because behind the scenes no one truly knows of your struggles, and in those moments, I honestly did not think I would make it. But I attempted bravery, and I look back now and think of those experiences with gratitude, as they have shaped me into the powerful woman I am today. It is important to know, that just as the triggers of dark times can remind you of your weaknesses and sorrow, they are also reminders of faith, love, hope and resilience. Now, at times when I stumble and fall again, I do so with compassion and understanding.

Years have passed and life today has so much more meaning, with two beautiful sons who have provided me with the true essence of life. I know if I would have gone to a place of no return on those fateful nights, I would never have experienced the joy that life has to give, which I so lovingly deserve.

I take both my sons' hands, as they walk on either side of me, on the soft sheet of white sand under our bare feet. We have come to take in the setting sun as we do frequently. I feel the salty air gently brush my lips and I can taste its embrace. The sea breeze blows against my face, welcoming me to be at one with its rhythm and flow. The sun is setting now into the Indian Ocean and soft pastel hues of pink, purple and blue fill the evening sky. As the sun sets deeper into dusk, the colours in the sky become richer and suddenly vibrant shades of orange, pink and red emerge creating a golden glow as far as the eye can see. The sky is reflecting onto the sand as the tide has turned, creating a mirroring effect as if heaven were on earth. There is an unforgettable ambience seeping below the skin, extending soul deep.

My sons run ahead laughing and playing. The salty sea is flat and calm as if I could simply walk on it. I feel at one with the universe, and I sense its power as the tide draws in and then out further again pulling the slightest of worries away. I stand still and take in a deep breath of life-giving air that flows through my body in exhilaration. Miracles and endless joy flow to me with every breath. The calmness and serenity I once cried for is here. I see my reflection on the wet sand, with the background of the most magical and breathtaking sky above me. I am now a goddess of light and love standing in unison with mother earth below me. I feel the loving connection of the universe and I graciously gain triumphant joy in the love that sits in my heart and the gentle fire in my belly. This time the fire is not raging out of control. It is not there to burn me or cause me pain, it is there to show me my light, my truth and my hope.

My boys come racing back to me and I welcome their loving embrace. I instantly discover an amazing sense of empowerment in not only realising that I can be love, but I can create love and that love can sustain and fulfil me for the rest of my days.

We casually stroll further down the beach before deciding it's time to go home as the full moon starts to rise on the opposite side of the sky. They both say, 'mum we love you to the moon and back' and I tell them I love them with all my heart and soul throughout the universe and all the galaxies that will always connect me to them for all eternity.

The Full Moon in all its glory represents a powerful energy in the universe, one that offers us clarity, focus and a deeper connection to our feminine energy. It is in the presence of this full moon that all of the world's wisdom comes to me and I am finally able to shed the pain of the past. 'What is this wisdom and your final message?' you ask. To always believe in your heart of hearts that you are the most important person in your life, and you are worthy of your own love. You can claim your power, embody your truth and celebrate it with acceptance and love. You can be the truest, most authentic version of yourself in each moment of every day without guilt, shame, or pain. In loving yourself you will become a magnetic force that will bring forth unlimited abundance, prosperity, and love into your life. And just as I tell my sons every day, before you attempt to love anyone else, remember to love yourself first and foremost. You have one precious life – you owe it to yourself to love thyself because life is too short not to. You have the power in you.

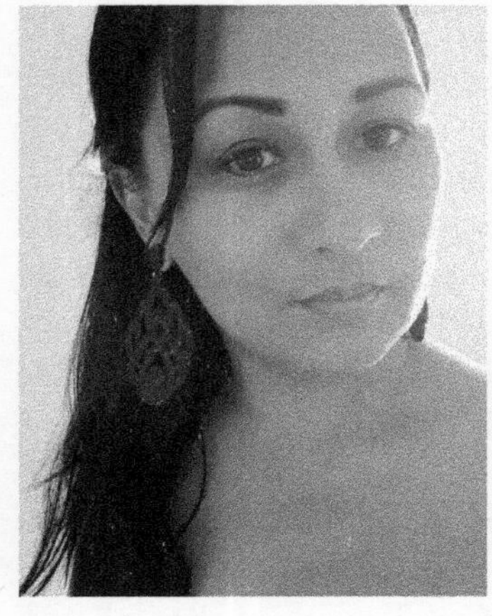

Niniella Marie

Hi, my name is Ninielia Marie (aka Nini Mills). I am a saltwater woman from the pristine turquoise waters of the Kimberley coast of Western Australia. My home by the bay is full of blossoming frangipani trees, touched by tropical weather, surrounded by beautiful white beaches and the most magical sunsets you will ever see.

I have come from humble beginnings but have created an amazing life of freedom, prosperity and wealth in its truest sense fostered through meaningful connection and creativity.

My greatest life purpose is raising my two beautiful sons. I am a proud Aboriginal woman, mother, leader, author, public speaker, life coach and mentor.

I love to tap into my creative flow which is a true reflection of my inner self and as such I thoroughly enjoy creative writing, interior design, fashion design, art, and photography.

As a life coach and mentor, I am a strong advocate for women's empowerment and am passionate about smashing through glass ceilings whilst also creating opportunities for other women to develop their capacity to lead the way for future generations.

My professional career has always focussed on advocating for and supporting the rights and interests of Aboriginal people. I have over 15 years' experience in Senior Management and Leadership and have held professional roles in government agencies at both Federal and State level and within community organisations focused on leading strategic direction, policy reform, program design and service delivery within the Indigenous Affairs sector.

I am a successful woman who has developed the power to manifest everything my heart desires. It is through my personal journey and my inherited wisdom that I hope to inspire other women to honour and love themselves so that they can also turn their dreams into reality.

With love,
Ninielia Xx

Email: ninieliamarie@outlook.com.au & ninielia2014@gmail.com

Lineage

Querida Perina

"We do the work our forebears were not able to – through circumstance or will. They have set the scene for us to continue." ~unknown

It didn't feel anything like an orange, sticking that needle into the pale, dimpled flesh of my mother's abdomen, despite the nurse's assurances less than a week earlier. Mum's breath held in silent anticipation, waiting expectantly for this moment to be over in her dimly lit bedroom. I knelt by her bedside, no room for hesitation now, and willed my hands to steady, my own breath to flow as I carefully, slowly, emptied the contents of the syringe into her chemical ravaged body.

Mum had been diagnosed with the big C at the beginning of that year. This moment, somewhere in the fog of days and weeks and months that followed in a daze of appointments, doctors, vomit, fear and my final year of high school, stands out sharply focused, never to be forgotten. It was one where I called on something from inside that my 17-year old self was not consciously aware she possessed. A strength, a courage and a grace, held unshakably deep within.

***

I will never forget sitting in the kitchen a few months prior, just shy of my seventeenth birthday, when Dad spoke the words no parent ever wants to speak and no child ever wants to hear.

"Mum has cancer."

I felt like the floor dropped away beneath me. The stool I had been comfortably and safely sitting on suddenly became the most treacherous place to be, resting on the edge of a deep, dark precipice – what I can only describe as the void. I now knew what it was to have your whole world turned upside-down in a moment.

Self-preservation and logic kicked in as Dad started speaking of the practical realities of what lay ahead – what type it was (aggressive), how advanced it was (very), what chance the doctors gave of survival (low), and how the only treatment (intensive chemo) may also be the thing that actually killed her.

I toppled over the edge at this point, spinning uncontrollably through that void, on the inside at least. Because it was clear there was no place for expressing emotions here amongst this logical, practical talk. I was well-versed in pushing emotions down after years of experience, denying my unwelcome 'negative' ones. "Good girls don't shout / cry / fight" was the message I received over and over; a coarse thread woven through my childhood that felt like an itch my highly sensitive and emotional self couldn't scratch. When I was younger these stifled feelings appeared in outbursts of anger, screaming and tears. When they became too big for my little body to carry any longer, the dam of withheld feelings broke its walls to overflow. I would numb myself as a young adult, unable to get away with emotional outbursts any longer and these feelings shape-shifted into deep depression that nothing could penetrate.

I swallowed my emotions down, landing back at the kitchen table with what felt like a thud. Afraid if I started crying I might never stop. I heard my own voice as though coming from somewhere distant calmly asking, "So, when does it start?" as I gulped down the fear, uncertainty and restless anxiety bubbling within. Any remnants of the little girl in me swallowed into that void.

***

I was sitting in Mrs. Cavanagh's classroom about a month after Mum was diagnosed, a good friend by my side. She was the one teacher at school who I felt I could turn to now. I'd been having trouble focusing on my schoolwork since Mum's diagnosis and as it was my final year, reached out for help.

The chalkboard had remnants of what looked like junior maths on it. Coincidentally, that was when Mrs. Cavanagh had first been my teacher. She had that open, warm and approachable, motherly vibe about her. I remember a time one of the boys in my Year 8 class absentmindedly began his question with "Mum?" before catching himself and trying to correct it. But it was too late. We'd all heard, and the whole class burst out in laughter, each of us silently and simultaneously breathing a sigh of relief that it wasn't us that had made the deadly social faux-pas. Though I'm sure it wasn't the first or the last time she'd heard that in her teaching career.

As I sat in the empty classroom with my teacher and my friend, the dam finally burst, tears flowing, as tissues were gently placed in front of me. My friend spoke the words I was unable to. I heard Mrs. Cavanagh's reply, thick and muffled as though the sound was travelling through the flood of my tears, before hitting my eardrum with a dull thud.

"It's going to be okay. I will notify the office and your other teachers, and you can apply to have the circumstances considered if it affects your results this year. There's nothing to worry about."

Her kind eyes looking straight into mine, her hand gently patting my arm, sending waves of concern and empathy into my being. It was the first time since Mum was diagnosed that someone had been primarily concerned with me in it all, with how I was handling it, with what support I did, or didn't have, at school and at home. For the first time, someone was willing and able to identify, and deal with, the fallout, not just the blast. Mrs. Cavanagh was my earliest example of what it was to 'hold space' for another being in their pain and suffering, and that there was nothing to be frightened or ashamed about in simply living this human experience; an example that served me well in the coming years.

***

"I don't care what the doctor says, you don't need someone messing around in your head," Dad stated emphatically at dinner one night, not long after Mum had begun chemo. He was referring to the doctor's recommendation that Mum consider seeing a counselor to support her with the impact that her cancer diagnosis and chemotherapy might have on her mental health.

"No way," Mum concurred, in full agreement with Dad's seeming disdain for the mental health profession.

My fork froze momentarily somewhere between the plate and my mouth. The inner turmoil and swirling thoughts I had been experiencing since Mum's diagnosis had me silently judging them for being closed-minded. An inner voice of deep wisdom inside me was certain there must be some benefit in looking at more than just the physical impact of this illness, and that undergoing chemotherapy was emotionally challenging. But it was something we never spoke of, and I knew better than to ask.

***

Mum and I sat in the pale waiting room of the family GP's office, outdated magazines scattered on the table. It was twelve months after Mum had completed chemo and been given the all clear that there was no more cancer in her system. My inner turmoil, though hidden during her treatment, remained unresolved and had transformed into depression. We were at the doctor's for me this time.

I finally heard that inner voice again saying, "I don't want to be here."

We were called into his office, and Mum told the Doctor why we were there. He nodded and made a few affirming noises.

"Just take these and you'll start to feel better in a few weeks," he stated calmly, matter-of-factly, as he handed me a script for anti-depressants.

"How long do I take them for?" I managed to ask quietly.

"For the rest of your life. Your brain isn't making the chemicals it needs to so you'll take these to do that for you."

That voice felt weaker now from being shuttered away, unwelcome, but still managed to tug at me, whispering, "No. I don't want to. There's got to be another way."

I brushed the voice aside. Lost, frightened and well trained to follow orders and hand over my power, I began taking the anti-depressant medication. Like clockwork. Every. Single. Day.

The complete numbness that ensued, while I can acknowledge was needed for a time of reprieve from the incessant, negative talk in my own head, eventually became more unbearable that the talk itself.

Cautiously, after eighteen months taking the medication, that inner voice took her chance again.

"It doesn't have to be this way," she whispered.

Listening, and after a long consideration, I slowly began to wean off the drug. The anti-depressant had ensured I was spared from the lowest of lows, but had also stolen from me even the slightest of joys, as it cocooned me into such a narrow sliver of feeling and expression that I no longer recognised myself.

Yet inside that cocoon, the incessant talk had simply been muffled so that I was unable to hear it. Stopping the medication was like taking off industrial grade earmuffs. The negative self-talk was still there, and had been there the whole time, even if I had stopped hearing it for a while thanks to the medication.

I didn't want to admit it, but by only taking medication, I'd been treating the symptom and not the cause of the depression, just like I had judged Mum for when she refused counseling during her chemotherapy. Over the next year and a half, I spiraled down deeper and further into depression than I knew was possible. What had previously been waves of negative talk inside had become a tsunami after being held back for so long by the meds.

I couldn't hide my inner state like I had the first time. Every aspect of my life and every relationship in it was affected and infected by the rancid relationship

I had with myself and my inner world. Every emotion I'd pushed down and denied didn't stop existing, but had rather festered and decayed into a pool of bitterness until I felt like a shell of the person I had known myself to be. For a time, I even forgot what it felt like to smile, convinced my facial muscles had atrophied, my entire world felt so blank and so bleak.

Thankfully life had other plans for me than to just give up and numb out on medication again. My housemate's girlfriend, a psychology student who was fighting her own inner battles, brought the medicine I truly needed. She told me about a therapist who came highly regarded.

"Yes," the inner whisper croaked, hoarse from being drowned out for so long. "This. This is the way forward," she nudged.

I had accumulated layers and layers of learned beliefs. I believed it was not acceptable or necessary to seek help for my emotional realm, and had a distrust of those who offered such help. So listening to my inner voice didn't come easily.

The therapist was masterful at creating a safe and supportive environment. Despite my initial resistance in that clinical, yet welcoming room, she equipped me with skills for day-to-day life. She encouraged me to take bold steps into territories (both inner and outer) that had previously been off-limits on my own.

I began taking a different type of anti-depressant in consultation with the therapist. Thankfully these ones didn't numb me out so much, and along with the inner work I did, the meds helped me trust the ground beneath my feet again and supported me in finally learning to swim through the waves that I had previously been drowning in.

Through it all, she was the one place I allowed myself to be supported. The one place I talked freely and openly. The one place it felt safe to do so.

Despite my racing mind, the mindfulness practices I learnt became a lifeline and anchor for me. I still carry these tools with me and call on them today when needed. I'm better able to hear the whispers of that little voice when I pay attention to the smooth, soft inhale that calls me inside my body, and the calm, steady exhale that grounds me there.

I stopped treating only the symptom of depression by exploring my inner world. Over time I've been able to approach its cause by practicing mindfulness and other skills learnt along the way.

I can see now that the depression came about because unconsciously, I had been trying to do all the 'right' things. I was living by my perception of other people's hopes and dreams for me, by other people's values, having no idea of what my own hopes and dreams were, or that I could even dare to have them.

***

I was sitting in another waiting room, this time thirty-one years old, starkly different to the one my family GP had consulted from. As I walked on the dark carpeted floor into the gynecologist's office, the heavy teak furniture towered ominously over me; a not-so-subtle message of who was in charge here and where the power lay.

I'd been experiencing increasing pain around my period along with a host of other related symptoms, and my current GP had referred me for a pelvic ultrasound to investigate.

After a brief greeting, the gynecologist impassively reviewed the scan results.

"You have an endometrioma on your right ovary. Do you want to have children?"

I was single and couldn't know that in less than two years I would meet my soul mate, best friend and life partner. Through my shock at his abruptness I replied timidly, "Um, not right now?"

"Then there's nothing that needs to be done. Just leave it. Come back and see me if you want to have a family."

He'd given me a brief and clinical explanation of what an endometrioma was, but did not discuss how it may be impacting my quality of life, or any follow up material for me to understand the future implications on fertility.

It was clear the appointment was over as he shut my file and glanced towards the door. Lost for words, and any sense of authority over my body, I stood and walked out of the room. Waves of shock and relief washed over me simultaneously.

I left, tail between my legs, with a sense of being broken and of holding a shameful secret deep in my womb that I was powerless to do anything about. The doctor's uninformed message brought me some misguided relief; I could pretend this diagnosis wasn't anything to worry about and just get on with life, which I readily did for another six years.

***

"B-b-but …" the single word barely escaped my lips, my head slowly shaking, my eyebrows furrowed in a frown of incomprehension, tears streaming down my face and yet I'd never been clearer and more certain of anything in my life.

I didn't know what to expect from the personal development seminar I attended about a year after walking out of the gynecologist's office. Sitting in a room of people who looked just as stunned as me, I'd spent the previous two days learning how my perception and judgements had created a one-sided story where I was the victim of my life's experiences.

I sat in the chair being guided through the Equilibration Process. This series of simple questions showed me the other side of my story. My conscious mind frantically searched for proof of how I'd been thinking for so many years, right up until an hour ago. It wanted proof of the story I'd been telling myself, of the judgements I'd made of my Mum, yet found nothing but perfection wherever it turned.

My mind expanded and heart exploded as I understood that everything Mum did had been perfect, as had everything that her mother did and her mother before that. Everything I'd been judging Mum for was perfect as well, and had led me to find the qualities I needed within myself to handle my life's experiences.

Thanks to listening to that little voice I now know as my intuition, I can look back on the day Mum refused counseling differently. I had been judging her for being closed to her emotions. Now I realise, that her refusal to look inside, became my driving force to do just that. Her discomfort in the emotional realm ensured it became the landscape I felt most at home in. And because of this, I am where, and who I am today.

I sat back in my seat, my mind truly quiet for the first time since hearing Dad share Mum's diagnosis in the kitchen almost fifteen years earlier. I saw all the events in my life and the people in it, who I was still telling myself a story about. In that moment I knew I needed to learn the Equilibration Process. Thankfully, life heeded my call, and the next steps to living my dharma, my calling, appeared through learning and facilitating the very process that allowed me to see the full picture.

***

Sitting on my couch, needle poised at the ready, I have a flash of certainty. All the pieces falling into place.

My partner and I had begun fertility investigations eight months earlier, after over twelve months of trying to start our family with no success. I'd been feeling conflicted about whether to start IVF treatment, recommended because of the progression of endometriosis diagnosed and dismissed all those years ago, or to opt for a natural holistic approach.

The IVF medication is self-injectable at home. When I learnt this a few weeks prior to that first injection, both paths lay out before me, neither more right or more superior than the other. I flashed back to my seventeen year-old self, holding the needle in Mum's dimly lit bedroom, and I knew with complete clarity and certainty that I had everything I needed within me, whichever path I chose.

I can now recognise that it's not about the path I take, but about going on the journey. Mum took the right path for her, and I'm taking the right path for me. I've said yes to some of the doctor's recommendations, and no to others, as I tune in to my body and its needs, connecting to my inner authority and strength. I did it when I came off anti-depressants, and I've done it again now, choosing to use holistic therapies hand-in-hand with conventional medicine and standing up for myself in the midst of it all.

Now as I find myself on my own medical path, I reflect back on Mum's journey – how she discovered she had cancer, the conversations we had around the kitchen table, and the seemingly never-ending doctor's appointments. In not denying the truth of my emotions and listening to my inner voice, I've come to recognise that Mum simply operated in a different way from me. I've come to find peace and acceptance through loving and not judging our differences.

Only with an adult perspective and my own medical journey, can I recognise how strong my Mum actually was, and the inner well she drew on to keep going, day after day, week after week and month after month, during her treatment and beyond. I can see the power within her to surrender fully, to withdraw from others, so that she could give to herself for the first time in her life. And she did this even though it went so strongly against the deep conditioning of women and mothers to put everyone else's wants and needs first. She was breaking patterns, lineages and cycles, and teaching me to do the same, preparing me for the journey of motherhood. I am now a continuation of that unfolding journey.

Without every event that had seemed lacking, and had those events happened any differently, from Mum's dismissal of counseling to my first gynecologist's sparse advice and beyond, I wouldn't be here now, with precisely what I need inside to deal with it all. I wouldn't be here now, clearing and closing this long-standing line of held trauma from the women in my family. I wouldn't be here now, doing the work that no one who came before me has done. I wouldn't be here now, clearing the way for those who follow.

Only now can I see that it's not just generational traumas that we inherit, but also generational strengths. Each and every injection I made, I did with the strength, courage and grace that I learnt from Mum all those years ago. I knew that I could do this because I already had. The mother in me was woken decades ago in that dimly lit room.

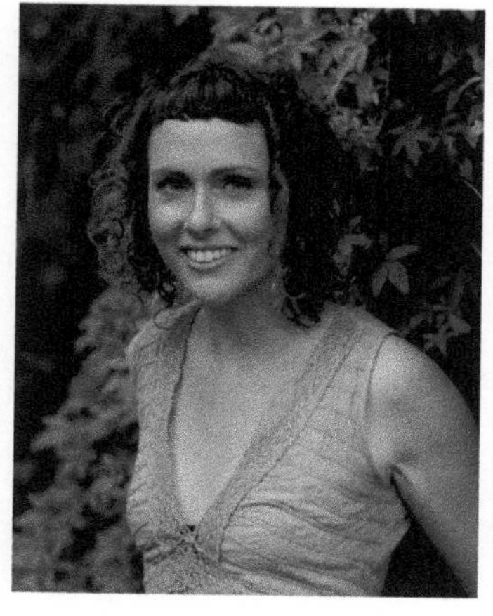

Querida Perina

I'm Querida, a no-nonsense, freedom-loving, heart whisperer whose superpowers include lovingly challenging your beliefs and perceptions to get you out of your head and into your heart.

To put a label on it, you might call me an Intuitive Body-Mind Guide. I call on a synthesis of the diverse learning's and experiences in my life from mindfulness, yoga and energy healing, to neuroscience and even my original degree in biology!

Unafraid to have the conversations that matter, the uncomfortable gritty ones, the scary ones that bring a sense of 'Can I really say/do/be THAT?' my innate curiosity has brought me to a deeper understanding of myself and ever closer to the truth of who I am by uncovering the stories and unconscious beliefs running behind the scenes, to connect with the inner wisdom and intuition housed in my heart and womb.

Born and raised in a small town on Australia's east coast, I spent much of my young adult life exploring this wide country and the world, learning from different cultures and absorbing experiences that have shaped my perception of life. Simultaneously, traveling the inner world for almost two decades has given me a steady compass, which I use to guide you in exploring your own inner world, learning to confidently swim and diving deep into the core truth of you.

I believe in finding simplicity in life, whether that be external (yes, I live in an actual tiny house on wheels), or internal by cutting through the stories we tell ourselves that make life more complicated than it needs to be.

I love nothing more than supporting and guiding you to your centre, where you too can leave behind the complex mind-chatter and tap in to that little voice that whispers as a clear, succinct knowing.

www.intuityou.com
Instagram: @intuit.you
Facebook: intuityou

Pandora's Box

Rachel Carmichael

My year 12 English teacher would always say that cliches had no place in good writing.

'Write something profound,' she would say to me. 'Your writing is like a momentary glimpse into your soul, don't waste your voice on some old, white man's cliché!'

Her voice has echoed in my head each time I have sat down to write this, as I'm not really sure where to begin when telling the story that is trapped in my soul bursting to escape. She was the first person to ever challenge me to seek out my power and bask in it, deservedly. And as I sit here contemplating the story desperate to breakout, I am reminded of another time where words pushed at my teeth and my jaws clenched to keep them inside. And how without that moment, without that decision to open my mouth and speak, no matter the consequence, I would be writing a very different story here today. Or perhaps not telling one at all.

***

'What are you thinking?' It was a simple enough question, but I knew that answering it would cause ripples in my life that had the potential to turn into a tidal wave, and I was terrified that wave might swell up and drown me. It was an uncomfortably hot day, my skin was sticky from sweat and my breathing felt shallow, as if it were catching in my throat with each exhale. I knew my silence wasn't going to be accepted for long, but I persisted at staring at my feet as they pawed the cold tiles and I willed the rest of my body to cool down too. A reassuring hand gripped my forearm gently pressing for an answer caught just behind my teeth.

'It's like opening Pandora's Box,' I responded slowly and with caution. 'Once I let out what's inside I can't ever put it back in, and you might not like what it is you are trying to let out.' I had hoped at the time that my own apprehension would be enough to curb the curiosity, but as I looked up from my feet, the eyes staring back at me were intensely fixed, no sign of nerves and no chance of wavering. My very own Pandora, and I was about to give her a key to all the things locked in my soul; things hidden away for my own protection (or so I had taught myself to believe). The key to a lock, that upon opening, would throw my world into chaos.

'You really want me to open it?' One last chance to back out, one last moment where retreating to the safety of familiarity, routine and 'normal' was still an option. But her eyes remained fixed on mine. There was something oddly comforting in their intensity that I would grow to appreciate.

'Sometimes, I wish we were more than just friends.' The words stumbled out of my mouth and sounded even more ridiculous than they had in my head. And with them came a wave of feelings and thoughts that I had not prepared myself for, each more confusing than the last, fear, guilt, relief, sadness, pain, excitement, each wave stronger than the last, and brutally bashing me against the sandbank that was my life up until this point. I think I knew in this moment, though it would take me months to accept, that the foundations of my adult life had been decaying for over a decade and that very soon, these waves would wash them away.

Pandora's face softened to a smile, half cheeky, half happy, a face I have since come to look for in my day for a sense of calm when all seems stormy. Her finger gently traced my arm in comfort. 'I already know that,' she said with a smile and then released my arm as our moment was interrupted. And it isn't really about that single moment. It isn't about kissing Pandora later that day, a mess of sweat and mango juice, and realising that what I was feeling wasn't completely one-sided. It wasn't about the lust or the desire that was overwhelming my every thought or the guilt and shame that quickly followed, propelling me back into silent confusion. It's about the months and years before that. Those moments of pleasure and trauma finally bubbling to the surface that had been shoved into a box and labelled, 'DO NOT OPEN.' Dealing with them would almost destroy me, but it would also set me free.

About a month earlier I had found myself woken from troubled sleep, sweating, crying, a ball of anxiety flooded with memories long since repressed. My husband lay next to me, though like he had for the longest time, he felt worlds away, asleep and wrestling with his own demons. As I lay there filled with sadness at how incredibly lonely I felt, a guilt niggled at me that I could not quite place. I was familiar with nightmares; they had haunted my sleep for most of my life. Many I had learned to accept and interpret through meditation and journaling, others were the remnants of PTSD continually suppressed and intentionally ignored. But this dream had been different. It danced silently across memories long since forgotten of a younger less inhibited Rachel, who wandered the world barefoot and fancy free, unchained by the expectations of the world, and unjaded by the people who would soon come to let her down. I watched her, this 14yr old version of myself, sitting on a roof hand in hand with my close friend. I was laughing hysterically and she was smiling at me like neither of us had a care in the world. And then the dream faded and I was catapulted back into my bed, a ball of confused emotion, crying silently into my pillow, hoping desperately not to wake my sleeping husband. 'Why have I forgotten this memory?'

It would be six months before I would realise the answer to that question, and another six before I would learn to truly understand and accept it. Twelve months that felt like a lifetime, twelve months that produced moments where I was completely broken. It was like tearing myself apart again and again trying to find the piece of me I hadn't even realised I had lost. My soul shattered to pieces a hundred times and I glued it back together a hundred and one, each time a little stronger and a little more powerful than the last. What I wasn't prepared for was the person I rebuilt to be someone completely different to whom I had expected.

She wasn't the Rachel who had spent most of her adult life chasing an idea of 'happily ever after,' looking for someone to choose her, to make her feel valid in existing. She wasn't the Rachel who stood joyous on her wedding day, unable to wipe the smile from her face, as she felt her life had become complete, crazy in love and full of hope for the future. She wasn't the Rachel who's heart broke and soul dimmed when she realised she may never have children, the Rachel that retreated away inside herself as she felt the failure of her body consume her. She wasn't the Rachel who watched helplessly as her happily ever after faded, no longer satisfied with ideals the world had preached to her, no longer safe in the idea that being a wife and a mother would make her whole. She wasn't the Rachel who had thrown herself tirelessly into work, day after day, hour after hour, desperately trying to prove to anyone, but mostly to herself, that her life had some kind of meaning or purpose. Nor the Rachel who watched her husband become a stranger she shared a house with; watching the loving companionship become obsessive co-dependency and longing to break free. No, the Rachel that emerged from the rubble and ashes of her crumbling-white picket fence life, was the essence of that laughing girl on the roof in the body of a woman, who suddenly remembered who the fuck she was, and remembered why, for almost two decades, she had hidden that memory under guilt and shame in the Pandora's Box of her soul .

There was nothing particularly unusual about that memory, it wasn't uncommon for us to meet on the train line that ran behind both our schools, talk about our days, sneak smokes and skip the class before lunch break. More often than not, we would find ourselves sitting on the roof of her house that backed onto the train line, watching the world spin by below us, laughing at our class mates caught up in the drama of high-school life. We felt so above it all. I don't know what made this day any different to the rest, but as we sat there on the roof, laughing and joking, for some reason it was different. I heard the distant sound of a school bell and sighed resting my head on her shoulder. She squeezed my hand. I laughed and then she kissed me, and then we both laughed again. That was the first time I ever kissed a girl. The second bell rang and we both jumped down from the roof and raced back in opposite directions back to school.

As a teenager I never understood the need to 'come out.' Most of my peers were idolised for their sexual conquests; the boys lorded over adding another 'notch to the belt' and girls desired they balance perfectly between innocent and experienced. None of them ever felt the need to explain, justify or announce their sexuality to the world, it simply was. And as far back as I can remember, I never could understand why. Why was it that if the person you had feelings for, sexual or otherwise, happened to be the same gender as you, your relationship or interactions now needed a label? A disclaimer that highlighted for the world – my relationship is outside the norm and is therefore strange, dangerous or less valid then someone else's. But even as a fourteen year old I was quick to learn that if you didn't fit into one of society's boxes, you'd be bent and broken until you did.

I am not sure how the story of the kiss on the roof became public knowledge, but by the next weekend it was a hot topic of conversation. I wouldn't say either of us were particularly bothered by it at first, it was easy enough to laugh off, two friends having a pash for fun, but as the weeks carried on and the jokes didn't end, I found myself avoiding secret smoko rendezvous on the train line out of fear of more talk. Everyone wanted to know 'what it mean,' and I don't think either of us had any idea what the answer was. So, we avoided the questions and eventually each other too. The situation all came to a head about a month later when a classmate called across the courtyard to me, 'so are you a dyke now?' I remember his words really jarred me; a. because I hadn't even thought about labelling myself before that moment, and b. because there was so much negativity and disgust in the way he asked it, the term still triggers a sick feeling in my stomach today.

I remember sitting in that courtyard in tears, friends trying to comfort me.

They all meant well but it wasn't really a situation any of them were equipped to deal with.

'You know that there is only one way to stop all the gossip Rach,' one friend commented. 'You just need to pick a side.' I stared at her blankly, a thousand thoughts pinballing across my mind in every direction. I didn't understand what she meant. Why were there suddenly sides to be on? Noticing my confusion another friend chimed in attempting to help. 'Here's the thing Rach,' he made his speech so matter-of-factly that I think it stuck in my subconscious for years after, 'It's ok if you're gay, its ok if you're straight, but you can't be both! Girls who kiss guys and girls are always just going to be seen as sluts who want the best of both worlds. So if you want the speculation to end, pick a side, stick to it and move on.'

I don't regret what I did next, or at least, not the actions I took. But looking back now I can see that this day started, not just a bad habit, but a belief system in me that would filter through every aspect of my existence. The man with whom I shared my sexual debut, was exactly that; a man, most likely with a wife, possibly children and a whole other life that I did not know nor care anything about. He protested a little, and I insisted a lot, and we fucked on a desk. It was decidedly average, slightly uncomfortable and in all honestly, over before I had much time to think about it. I returned to the world of gossiping teenagers, 'officially straight' and as quickly as the rumours had begun they soon dried up. But now rather than being the possibly queer skank, because I had kissed a girl without first aligning myself with a sexual identity, I was a sought after commodity; 'Experienced, but not slutty.'

That wouldn't be the first time I would have my value decided by my interactions with a man. And while I still feel the experience was completely in my control, and my decision to enter the sexually active world in an attempt to prove my questionable sexuality seemed reasonable at the time, I wish someone had been there back then to tell me that sexuality, especially female sexuality, is so much more than who you fuck. I wish someone could have told me that it was ok to kiss your friend on the roof and ok to fuck a guy on his desk, and ok to have all the experiences that came after that, and still not 'pick a side.'

By the time I was eighteen I had locked that memory so far down in my subconscious and thrown away the key, I had almost forgotten it. Forgotten what it was like to feel threatened by the people around you, forgotten what it was like to have your peers talk about you and shame you into silence, forgotten that I had chosen peer acceptance over the girl on the roof and essentially ended our friendship, forgotten what it was like to feel who you are is defined by one moment, one action, and that you would have to live with that forever.

I wish my next time learning this lesson had been as easy to forget.

Unlike the memory on the roof, when I look back on this day I can remember everything. I remember exactly what I was wearing, down to the bra and undies, perhaps because they ended up in an evidence bag. I can remember exactly how much I drank; one cruiser and half a warm beer. Probably because I was asked over and over again in a police interview room if I was sure I wasn't drunk this night. I can remember the last song I heard in the bar, Eagle Rock, probably because I later sung it to myself on repeat in my head to block out the sound of their voices, laughing and egging each other on. I remember the buckle of my belt scratching me as it was forced open by multiple sets of hands. I remember the taste of dirt mixed with tears from the garden bed I passed out in trying to get away. To this day I still wake up screaming some nights, coughing up what I think is dirt. And I remember the terror, the complete and utter helpless fear I felt, when I was carried by my wrists and ankles, a limp, drugged mess, back to the car for it all to start again.

But those details are not the part of the memory that defined me. So much of the trauma I still carry with me from that night has nothing to do with what physically happened. It was the aftermath that truly destroyed me. It was the responses of the people around me that would once again shame me into silence. My boyfriend at the time, who rapidly evacuated our relationship in the days following my rape, asked me if I had cheated on him and was just using this as a story to cover it up. My friends, so desperate to not rock the boat made comments like, 'it's not like you're exactly innocent Rachel, maybe you gave them the wrong idea.'

I lost count of the insensitive things police officers said to me during the investigation process, but the one that sticks out most was a senior detective in the Sexual Assault Unit who remarked, 'young girls these days think it's helpful to report every rape and sexual assault that happens, when really it just makes it harder for us to investigate the important ones.' I'm not even sure what he meant by it. What makes a particular rape more important than another?

But the comment that did the most damage, the one that found its way into the depths of my soul, was an off-the cuff-comment my father made to me in a moment of drunken anger and frustration. 'This is why you have a boyfriend, to protect you from ending up like this, this never would have happened if you'd been out with a guy that night.' It is probably the most powerless I have ever felt in my life, and what made it worse was the sickening feeling that it had been my fault; that I had given that power away.

So with this idea in my head, this concept that I had set myself up for all that pain by simply having one night out with a girlfriend instead of a boyfriend, I began my next decade long mission of trying to fix myself, trying to mould and shape myself in the image of all the other girls around me. The ones whom

I had determined were succeeding at life, based on their ability to find a man and keep a man. Trying to make myself into the perfect girlfriend, perfect wife, perfect would-be mother, in the hope it would protect me from ever reliving the terror that comes from being an unprotected female member of society. Slowly over time, I etched away anything about me that was outside 'the norm.' I dulled the parts of me that made me different and fixated on making myself what other people wanted, in a delusional pursuit of security in sameness. I would fool around with women, but I only ever dated men. I am pretty certain I even broke a girls heart once who dared to risk the 'straight' status I was clinging to. To be honest I think it broke my heart a little too. And with every layer I tore away, my power dwindled and my sense of self faded into nothingness, buried in a box with the girl on the roof.

When I met my husband, I was probably at one of my lowest points. I think we genuinely needed each other as much as two people possibly could, and we found comfort and then love in the mutual needing. It was everything I had spent years looking for; someone to come home to each night, someone to wake up next to in the mornings and when the nightmares came, someone to be there with you and love you and protect you from anything that could harm you. And for years that was enough. For the most part we presented to the world as the perfect married couple, and to be fair in many ways we were. We rarely ever fought, we had a nice collection of 'happily married' friends, we had a healthy and active sex life and we had all the same interests, every last one. So why was I waking in the middle of the night sweating about a secret kiss almost twenty years in the past?

I think the turning point came in the days after I found out that my husband and I would most likely not have children. We were both so broken by the news that it changed us as people in ways we couldn't see from inside our marriage. I remember feeling desperate for a purpose, for a reason that would help it all make sense. There had to be something else on the horizon for us, something else that was coming our way that would fill the hole this information had left us both with. But while I was out there searching for answers, seeking out the next adventure that I was sure was waiting to be found, my husband retreated into himself; a mix of self-pity and self-blame. So many nights I cried myself to sleep with the sheer weight of it all. I had done everything I was supposed to do, I had been exactly who society had told me to be. I had followed every fucking step and here I was awaiting the next one, and the ground had suddenly been pulled up from beneath me. I looked in the mirror and had no idea who it was staring back at me anymore.

Reclaiming my power happened slowly and some days I didn't even realise it was happening. Other days it felt like I went to battle for it and barely made it out alive. The scariest thing I have ever done was to admit to myself that the life I was living was no longer making me happy. I had spent two-thirds of my life convinced that I was broken and needed fixing, and then suddenly here I was realising that what was truly broken was the high school sex education system that let a teenage girl grow up thinking she was damaged for liking guys and girls. What was broken was the legal system that was rampant with victim blaming and brushing under the rug anything that was uncomfortable or messy. What was broken was patriarchal notion that women are born to be wives and mothers, and a failure to do that, was failing as a human. What wasn't broken was me. I was complicated – yes. I was controversial and non-conformist and all the things I had been told good girls shouldn't be. But I wasn't broken.

Writing this has been like opening Pandora's Box all over again and there were days where I thought it would break me, where I honestly couldn't see why my story mattered, or why it needed to be told. But then our due date came around, and I was sitting in a bar with my circle of women, Pandora sat next to me drawing circles on my palm and laughing as they compared their sexual identities without a care in the world, when one turned to me and said; 'You know Rach, we all get to do this, be exactly who we are and be totally ok with it, because you showed us it was ok by doing it first.' And somehow, without meaning to, I had become their Matriarch. We were all rising together, and I felt so fucking complete.

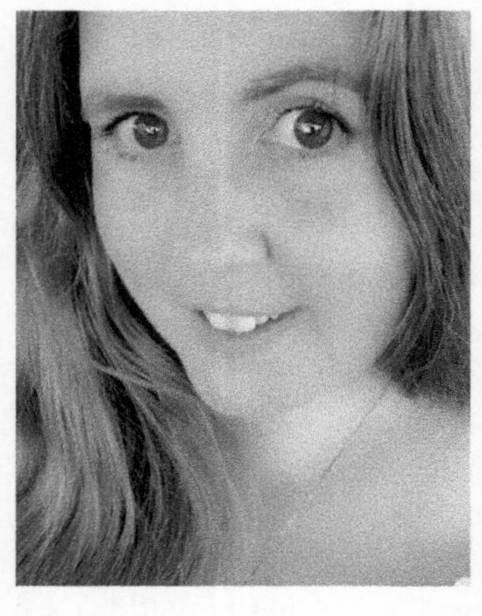

Rachel Carmichael

My name is Rachel Carmichael, and I am a daydreaming, moon gazing, nudity enthusiast living in the outer northwest of Melbourne.

Fiercely protective and at times overly empathetic, my day job sees me managing and coaching at a gymnastics club with the soul goal of fostering a safe and supportive place to learn for not just the 600 children that walk through the door every week but also the 30+ coaches, many of whom transition to adulthood during their time there.

At home my friends affectionately refer to me as "The Naked Witch on the corner" and my home alternates between meeting place, party house and short term accommodation for anyone who finds themself needing somewhere to go, and isn't adverse to the "bowls of rocks" or jars of feathers found on every surface.

In the same way many have found sanctuary in my home, from a young age I found my place of comfort in writing. From youthful fantasy told to my eager friends on the playground, to poems and songs my school teachers censored for fear of their honesty, writing was my outlet. At University I majored in English Literature and Philosophy and it was there that I learned how powerful it can be to share your soul with a stranger through writing. I have filled pages with words on days when I could barely speak and though I never had an audience in mind, without meaning to one found me.

I am passionate about the voices of all those who identify as women being heard and have contributed to and advocated for the #letusspeak movement as well as nominating my club as a safe space for LGBTQI+ members as part of the Pride Cup.

I believe every woman has a story to tell and that in sharing those stories we are paving the road for all those that follow.

Rach xx

Instagram: @the_nakedwitch
Facebook: thenakedwitch

Lifeless

Rebecca Lee

I found my tribe when my body was lifeless. Yes, my heart was beating but my spirit was long gone. I felt the Matriarch's of my circle cling to my spirit body while it was submerged in a muddy quicksand. The women gifted muffled whispers, 'you are worthy.' They continued their life-giving breath until I could find the belief. It was such a delicate and lengthy process.

Only a decade earlier I had danced as a youthful girl, tip-toeing on the earth with freedom and weightlessness of non-attachment. Opportunities were bountiful. I was oblivious to the lurking demons that would form within me.

I met the love of my life as I rippled freely in my late 20's, or so I thought at the time. Hindsight is so bittersweet. We embarked on the picket fence journey, hand in hand. Blindly waving goodbye to youth and individuality of our own sovereignty.

The day of settlement came. We strolled up the driveway, presenting ourselves to the future and our newly-purchased home. Can you fucking believe it? The keys from the real estate wouldn't open the front door. For real! The commencement of a landslide.

It was supposed to be the pinnacle, our bearing of children. Creation of the new generation. I was gifted with a transition to motherhood. Whilst we had been blessed with fertility, all else around us slowly decayed and declined.

We fed our children with every drop of time, only ever nourishing their beautiful souls. They were everything, the centre of all universes. The arrival of children combined with intense focus on them, gave birth to our shadow sides. It triggered feelings of anxiety, fear, doubt, and uncertainty, about the world, our parenting and relationship. Trust, respect, intimacy, communication; all the foundations of our once healthy relationship became lost in the blur of everyday living. He could no longer understand me and I could no longer calm his storms. We lost the ability to love each other.

I felt this foundational shift unravel over time. It revealed a vast expansion of distance between two opposites. As I felt the magnitude of our accumulated failures bare down upon us, I withdrew into myself. I surrounded my heart with concrete walls. In closing off, I let the volcanos of pain erupt silently within me for many years. It was so toxic, an inability to be expressive of my suffering. It commenced destroying resilience and belief in self-worth.

I could equally see an internalised turbulence in his eyes, and try as I may, I could not reach him. Yet I always trusted in and felt our love for each other. Even now, I know this was so.

With distance formed, comfort was found in the arms of another lover. Society dictates that to land in that space, is a treason of the heart, but my thinking on that was challenged. I found myself contemplating the concept of monogamy.

I sought understanding. Not just of alternative relationship dynamics. I sought understanding to offer acceptance of my life partner. I sought forgiveness for mistakes that had been made by both of us.

I reflected on all the ways we had both closed off from each other and how I had contributed to pushing him away. I found ignorance in belief that a soul would not crave intimacy from another during a lifetime. To deny that need and to have an inability for freedom of expression and exploration was to feed further distance.

My lover and I finally had an opportunity to close our distance. We trialled permission to accept each other's flaws. I asked for a declaration to values of trust and respect. A sharing and acceptance of our rawest truths. After many years of silence we found each other again, passionately, for the briefest moment.

Yet the affection soon dwindled, we reverted to living on auto-pilot. A darkness was exposed within me, it fed the devil. My soul was poisoned with the treason of secrecy and his lack of regard for my offering of unconditional love. We continued a frosty hiding of ourselves from each other. It was the final catalyst for my complete loss of self; my darkest days known on this earth, in this life. I was living with numbness and without joy. Perfectly balanced in ignorant awareness that I was stiflingly unfulfilled.

A loss of self is the most eerie feeling. It is not a depressive state, but intense feelings of absence and lack. I did not see the world in colour. The only reprieve was the grounding and laughter of my little people. I desperately wanted togetherness for my family. I kept sinking deeper into despair with a rational that togetherness was my children's ultimate source of happiness. I was anchored so deeply in my monotonous reality and prioritising my children.

Then one day I found a circle; a group of most incredible, empowering, non-judgemental women. I felt an immediate, yet minute, adjustment to the sails of my life vessel.

I sat in their presence weekly, for years. I introvertedly listened to them openly describe their pains, while I silently weaved mine into the art I created. We gathered together in the most sacred of spaces. It was a safe space, for stories to be told so that our shame could die and unheard burdens of life could be released.

One evening, the Matriarch of our group allocated an activity where we were encouraged to write ourselves a love letter. I could not find a single word. I had completely lost all value of myself. What the fuck? I left that night with page bare, and I felt completely broken.

Sometime later, on a very ordinary day, the most ordinary yet cynical, remarks were made by my partner. I can't even describe the switch in feeling, other than a penny drop. It opened a floodgate of emotion. I dragged every piece of his clothing from the room our children were created in, and discarded it all to the hallway. It was over.

It came from nowhere and with intensity; a sudden recognition that I was living my life with an absence of joy. A realisation that when my children tried to play with me, they never saw me smiling. An understanding that to simply live with physical togetherness of a family unit was of no life-giving value.

It became evident that the ultimate gift for my children was not in keeping the family together, but in being able to model happiness for them. I could not offer happiness in a place where my mind constantly spoke of internal sadness. Why am I not enough? Why can't I make this work? What more do I need to give? Why are we not working? It was time to acknowledge that we fuelled each other's own toxicity and self-doubt. It was time to walk away so that I could heal, and I gave myself permission.

We spent another 4 months living under the same roof, on an eggshell of silence. It was an all too familiar feeling. A reminder of the spark I felt missing. This time instead of sitting with pain, I allowed it to fuel my action and it shifted a gear. I started packing one box at a time, and took each day at a time, while I searched for new shelter.

One night when the kids were asleep, my ex and I sat at the kitchen table. We came together. It was the first time in many years we sat and looked each other in the eyes for an extended length of time. We both surrendered and dropped our guard. We spoke our deepest truths. We spoke of the ways we could share time with our children and how we could say goodbye. We made informal agreements and declarations of lifelong friendship. It was the togetherness we had been seeking for so long from each other and yet it was too late. We both felt free; free of the burden in knowing you are not enough for your lover.

Finally, I found a new roof. The first weekend my children spent at their old home, I returned to my humble rental. Upon closing the door, I sealed the locks to the world. I slumped on my uncomfortable second-hand couch for two entire days and nights, hardly moving. A wave of emotion fell over me that I had never lived through before. It was emptiness; a deep realisation of my lack of purpose and direction. I played and repeated the most aggressive music. It fed my numbness. No tears fell that weekend and I drank myself to oblivion.

I spent the next few months home-schooling my children. It was a genuine blessing in disguise. I re-established my roots to the earth and claimed my space in a new place. I learned to listen to my children's laughter without the constant feeling of hovering eyes, or a judgement of worthiness by another. I learnt to play with them again. I learnt to play. I was finding spirit. I was rebuilding.

I found the strength within myself to connect with another man. He offered a safe space to unashamedly speak of the ways we needed our bodies touched. We fucked and I had one of the most intense squirting orgasms of my life. I stepped out of thoughts of loss and found myself starting to question my individuality. For the first time in many years, I looked to the future and what I wanted it to hold.

I booked myself two nights away at the most extravagant of hotels; the best room with the best views. I spared no expense on the luxuries of life. I walked the riverbank, gathered sticks and stones with an empty mind. I swam in the pool on the coldest of days in the coldest of water. It was a baptism.

I felt refreshed and renewed. It was the final disconnect from the world and myself. Sitting amongst the plushness of my room, I felt a comfort in my isolation. I felt comfortable within myself. I finally wrote myself the love letter. I finally cried and it was gentle. I let tears fall to my cheeks as words spilled to the page. I reached out to my circle sisters, a Matriarch said, 'let the tears fall, feel what you need to feel.' Have truer words ever been spoken?

I vowed to love myself again. I made a commitment to accepting all my flaws and unashamedly sharing them with the world. I stepped into my power, remembered my truth and embraced the darkness of my shadows.

"You are a shining light guiding those on their path, and when your light dims, you know how to reach out to others and seek what you need.

"You are worthy …

"Of loving yourself.

"Of allowing the love of others to enter you.

"You have worked so hard to tap into your guidance system, your intuition.

"Trust it, follow it!

"Allow it to lead you to all the places you heart seeks.

"With love always."

When I finished writing, I sat in stillness and quite reflection of the decade. I found realisation that I had just journeyed through a lifecycle. A process of death and rebirth. You see, all cycles are underpinned by creation, birth, growth, ageing and death. All cycles have a summer, autumn, winter and spring. Light and dark, night and day. It's within all of us. Our body, mind, spirit and journey.

I finally awoke to the lesson. For me, embracing all stages of the cycle and facing the shadows, preparing for the winters, is the essence of being able to truly step into power through life's journey. I had lived in a winter, with silence. I had felt the crisp snow numb my skin. It made the new spring day extraordinary. I was no longer looking at life through a grey shade.

My stepping into power is in knowing I will land in another winter. Perhaps where my body will age and I will again question my worth. Perhaps it will be retched with a loss, grief or trauma. Who fucking knows what it will be, but I know it is coming.

You see I sit between two worlds now; I sit between my winters. I'm living in spring and feel a summer calling. I can once again feel myself tip-toe and move freely on the earth, flowing through life with self-reliance and a newfound resilience. I feel myself radiating, it speaks directly to and feeds my heart space.

This newfound knowledge evoked an explosion of thought within me; all of the longings that were too long supressed, a surge of creativity, passion and inspiration for all things in life. Thoughts of what I wanted as a person and a woman, not as a partner or mother. They are thoughts I had not visited for such a lengthy time.

I met another guy with the intention to just fuck, but in him I found a kindness. He listened to me for understanding and could hear my sadness. When our bodies came together, I found for the first time in my life that I was able to sit in a submissive space with a lover without feeling a pressure to please the other, without sitting in my own headspace and offering judgement to myself. In surrendering, I had expected to be devoured, but instead he offered such careful and gentle touches. We made love. It was magical and I felt happy.

It was a healing process for me, a revelation that I had lived in self-isolation for most of my life. My heart space had been forever surrounded by the guarding of walls, due to accumulated traumas. I had established patterns of ultra-independence, and over-reliance on self.

I had been in a constant cycle of refusing love, help and support from all sources. I know that I had pushed and driven away my life partner at the most critical times when I should have offered communication and transparency.

My walls were fed by self-doubt, engrained at some point along the precious timeline of life. They were built for constant protection, but were an icy deterrent to receiving love. To be open to pinnacles of love and happiness is to be vulnerable to pain, loss and failure. I was always sitting in fear.

It was time to live vulnerably with my heart space open. It was time to drop the guard. I no longer wanted to protect myself. I wanted to start taking risks and be open to accepting whatever should land on my path. It was time to break my own toxic patterns and cycles of behaviour. I will now happily live in the trenches, to live a life searching for treasures. Live a life seeking joy and rolling with the punches during the search.

I stand in my new-found power, ready to help lead women to a journey of their own discovery, a union with their voice and belief in self-worth. I need to continue sharing the wisdom and healing, and to pay my respects to the matriarch's that bestowed it to me. They kept the fire of my spirit burning while I no longer could. So I share my story, in an effort of permission giving to another woman.

Life is too short to have lack of respect for your own internal truth. Listen to your heart. Feel what you need to feel. This space feeds your intuition. Allow those messages to guide your decision-making and actions. The changes of the seasons come too quickly. Acknowledge your needs and desires. Allow yourself to live for what your heart seeks.

Find a space with a lover that makes you feel like you are dancing on the inside. Rest in that space. Let their love enter you and allow them to build you from your weaknesses. Allow them to be a refuge where you can share the raw abyss that swirls within you.

Allow non-judgemental women to encircle around you. They will help you hold the burden of your world. They will offer the comfort you seek. They will hold you in a safe and nurturing space, until you can heal and set your burdens free.

If you are barely tip-toeing, I say dance with one step at a time.

If you are tired of the way you are being fucked, guide the touch.

If you have lost yourself, find just one truth first.

Allow yourself to journey the healing process. When we heal and love ourselves we can radiate love to the world. Whatever it is that you do, do not let yourself completely drown in your winters. Yes, listen and learn from that place, but do not sit idle.

I recently became stranded interstate with border closures, and had the most marvellous human reach out to me: my children's father and my best friend. He knows my coldest winters and deepest darkness more than any other person on the planet. He offered to pay whatever it cost to fly us home to safety. He has stepped into his power as the most amazing protector and provider for our children, even after adversity.

I feel so blessed to have ventured a lifecycle with him. In learning to love ourselves first, we have learnt to care for each other again. We have finally learnt to love each other and have absence of all the heavy hatred.

I stand proud now, in a warrior pose, bare heart raised vulnerably to the sky. I keep my heart space open for myself first and foremost. I feel the confident sway of my body emerge as my womanhood flourishes. I feel a letting go of expectation and feel comfort to simply embrace all that flows to me. The people surrounding me have seen me come alive. I now move weightlessly, I am again dancing.

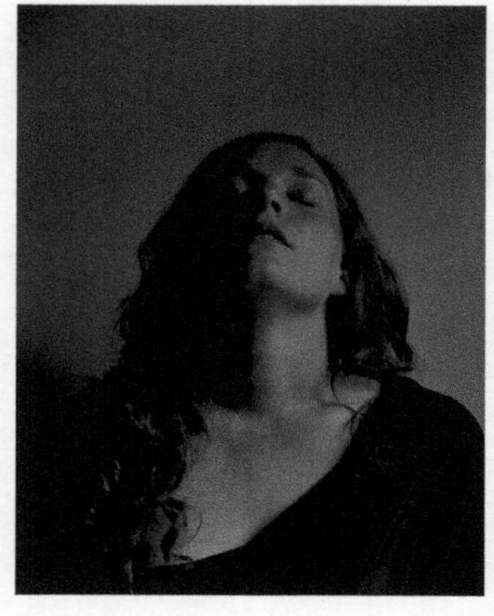

Rebecca Lee

I am a lover of word porn and its many forms.

Throughout my career, I have developed a sharp skill set of word mergement. Holding a bachelor's degree in business management, my profession requires report writing for an executive level audience. A boredom arose from this sterile, analytical writing genre. This gave me a catalyst for creativity.

In recent years, I transitioned to crafting words utilising a dialect of mystical realism. I have produced and shared a series of linguistic pieces online.

Highly introverted, I find writing to be the safest form of expression and communication. Key influences of my writing are connection to cultural practice or higher source.

Formally baptised into the Roman Catholic community, I have felt a disconnect to that theology for much of my life.

Profound influence for change was the emergence into daily life and religious practices in Japan, where I resided for nearly 2 years. The experiences of ceremony, ritual, chanting, and meditating opened a new world. A culture underpinned by Shintoism and Buddhist theology gave birth to my spiritual baptism.

I recently travelled a life altering path, meeting modern day Shamans, Tribal Matriarchs and powerful Circles of Women. I find a connection to spirit through earth medicine and ritual underpinned by indigenous cultures.

My writing draws on these influences and is now crafted to offer a bridge for reconnection with source. I believe in a world of cultural taboo, people are encouraged to disconnect from themselves and others in order to comply. I feel passionately that feelings and voices should not be muted. My belief is that written words are the echoes that ripple through generations.

To connect with my writing, publications, workshops and events, visit:
www.rebeccaleeauthor.com

A Descendent of Humble Beginnings

Sandra Erica

I descend from a long line of real life-warriors and leaders, humble yet victorious change-makers, unsung heroes, free spirited souls who lived life with the greatest of empathy and compassion for others. I feel a deep sense of pride for my ancestors who walked before me, and who inadvertently made me the person I am today. They each had a hand in creating and shaping my identity.

My parents instilled in me values of compassion, empathy, and inclusivity very early in life. I was taught to accept everyone regardless of how they looked, their cultural background, socio-economic status or the colour of their skin.

Both of my parents migrated to Australia from Italy. My father first arrived by ship sometime in the 1960's and spent ten years of his young life travelling the country before he returned to Italy where he met mum and together, they returned to Australia for a better life. It wouldn't be until I returned to the motherland just after my 21st Birthday that I would come to truly understand what they meant, when I would realise their humble beginnings and where they grew up, and when I would truly appreciate the history of my ancestors.

Growing up in the 80's I always remember our home being full. All of the neighbourhood kids would be at our place, virtually every day. We had a garage out the back, with a pool table and an old school video gaming table. It was like the youth centre our little community never had. I remember mum saying she'd rather have them at home where she knew they were safe.

I would eventually go on to become a youth worker. Coincidence?

When I stop and think, I realise we had enough as children. My parents provided for us exactly what we needed, everything we wanted and more, but they also chose not to spoil us – I believe they instilled in us, values and morals, passed on via our ancestors that will never slip away.

As a child I felt safe and protected. I felt a sense of security, protected not only by my parents, but also by my siblings and their many friends who frequented our home, and of course, a very large and extended Italian family. I had connection and identity. I belonged.

But during my first year of high school in the early 90's, **everything changed.**

I was bullied, picked on, teased and called horrible names. Mean boys said nasty things to me, and nasty things about members of my family.

I felt a deep sense of personal shame about the bullying, and I lacked the courage to actually admit to it, or openly talk about it (until now). Instead I tolerated it and spent many nights journaling my thoughts and feelings, as well as, many nights spent crying alone in my room.

I could never find my voice to tell those I loved most, the truth.

I was bullied, but never wanted my family to know. Maybe If I had opened up and been truthful with them, things may have played out differently. I know my parents would not have tolerated me being bullied, my brother and sister would have hurt ***anyone*** who picked on me, and their friends would likely have done the same.

I guess I felt a need to protect them the way they had always protected me. I didn't want them to be hurt by what I was going through, or hurt by the nasty things being said.

Part of the shame was me not wanting to let them down. In my mind I thought they would be disappointed in me; my young mind at the time not realising it wasn't actually my fault that other kids treated me so badly. I now realise, my family would never have been ashamed at all.

Some days all I wanted, was to die.

The bullying got so bad for me that I actually changed schools. I begged mum to let me transfer, telling her I hated going to a Catholic private school. I never told anyone the real reason for wanting to leave, which was to escape the incessant daily bullying.

Even after I left and moved on ready to start fresh at a new school with a new beginning, because let's face it, kids can be cruel, classmates at my new school had heard the rumours of what happened. Before I knew it, I was very quickly teased once again, bullied and made fun of; my new bullies had nicknamed me 'Flabanuda.'

I managed to get through high school ok, relatively unscathed. Eventually things got better. I made new friends. Aside from the normal teenage struggles (I won't downplay it, because life for young people is not easy), but things did get better. I had plenty of lows, but I also had many highs.

By the time I was fifteen, I had decided I was going down one of two possible career paths – one was youth work. I realised early in life through my own struggles, and those of others around me, that I wanted to help and work with young people. The other was film making. Yeah a part of me wanted the bright lights of Hollywood! But what I really wanted was to tell true stories about the reality of life for young people. Not to exploit them, or make money from their struggles, but to shine a light on the reality of life for them, to raise awareness and educate people to tell the truth.

Now like I said I was fifteen, so over the next few years, I changed my mind a million times about what I would do with my life. Even now in my forties I'm still working out what I'll be when I grow up.

In the end, I chose youth work. In the background and in my spare time however, I wrote many pieces – stories, screenplays and poems – but that became, at the time, what seemed an unrealistic and unachievable dream I pushed to the side.

My youth work career has been an incredible journey of self-discovery, personal learning, development and growth. I have been fortunate to work with amazing young people who have changed my life, and I have been mentored by some of the youth sector's greatest and best.

The best part? Along the way I met my now husband Dave, who shares my passion for youth work. Together we have been blessed to work in some of the most amazing places across Australia and with some of the most incredible people we will ever know.

I am incredibly grateful for everything we have seen, experienced, learned and lived through together.

We have never been the couple to ***conform with the norm:***

When we could have been at the peak of our night clubbing days, we chose late nights working with young people. While our friends were back-packing through Europe, we chose to live in Australia's own outback and roughed it in some of the country's most remote and isolated communities. We were engaged for six years before actually tying the knot, due to countless cancelled planned dates, opting instead to continue our outback adventures. We eventually chose a destination wedding on the beautiful shores of Vanuatu.

And when it came to, starting a family, instead of creating new life, we very consciously decided to 'foster' in hopes of providing a better life to children and young people in need. We have seen so much rejection, abandonment, grief and loss through our work, that we knew we would be a different kind of family. I never had a burning maternal desire in me to give birth, and I have always seen motherhood as much more than a biological connection.

By no means, has our journey been filled with butterflies, unicorns, fairies and rainbows – we've been through some hardcore, heartbreaking, life changing, next level shit (some of our hardest days, we are living right now).

But we've also been lucky to meet some of the most amazing people ever, and to be exposed to, welcomed and a part of Indigenous Australian cultural experiences like no other.

By far one of our greatest experiences to date, that we both still speak of and reminisce about, was our time, not only working, but living among and within remote Aboriginal communities in the Kimberley region.

Youth Work is not an easy profession, it takes a certain kind of person to do remote youth work. I'm not even talking a regional town here, but actual remote community, isolation, middle of nowhere, youth work is different again.

The youth work profession sets (necessary) rules and boundaries in order to protect ourselves and those we work with, but those boundaries have been developed by metro-based workers and so easily spoken of, yet are not truly reflective of the reality of life and work in a remote community, where you literally become a part of that community.

It becomes your home, they become your family, you are truly accepted into their space, they know where you live, they are your neighbour, they will protect and guard you for life, and they accept you as one of their own.

We were young and naïve when we first embarked on our remote youth work adventure, but we felt incredibly privileged and in awe of what we were seeing, doing and experiencing.

So many amazing memories, but just as many great times, were almost always coupled with times of grief, loss, and significant trauma.

Twenty-five – That is the number of people, a combination of young people we have worked with, friends, and family members – But twenty-five is also the number of people 'close to us' in some way, we have lost to suicide.

Twenty-five incredible humans who have forever left their imprint on our hearts, and who lost their battle with life.

Losing someone to suicide is one of the worst pains imaginable, And each and every time it happened, it would cut deeper than the last.

Someone told me recently they admired the strength, bond and love I have with my husband, despite all of our struggles, heart ache, grief, loss and trauma. They thought it was incredible we were still so strongly connected and in love. I had never before stopped and considered this myself, but it struck a chord with me. How true. I am incredibly fortunate to have found my soul mate and life partner in Dave. And together, despite all of our struggles, we have pulled through and continue to.

I'm a mother, and here is what I know: ***No family is truly perfect, because perfection does not exist.***

Our home is always full, just like it was when I was a child; it is forever filled with children, teenagers and young adults. It's full of laughter, joy, happiness, tears, sadness, anger, frustration, sibling rivalry that is next level (in so many ways), but most of all, it's filled with love. Unconditional love.

But while I see myself as a mother and feel the love a mother has for her children, I'm a different kind of mum.

I've never carried a child in my womb, I've never given birth, never breast fed a baby, never held any of my children in my arms after their birth, was never thrown a baby shower, or hosted a gender reveal party.

But it makes me no less of a mother.

The child protection system calls me a 'foster carer' (*insert eye roll), but I know I'm a mum.

I have been hurt by the thoughtless words of others too many times to count:

'But don't you want kids of your own?'

'Why do you do it?'

'Why would you choose to look after such damaged and troubled kids?'

'Aren't you worried how they might turn out when they are older?'

They ***are*** my own.

I do it because I believe it was my destiny to.

I do it because every child deserves love and family.

No, they are not damaged.

Doesn't every parent worry about their kids and what they will become?

But the comment that hurts most is when they have the nerve to say to me that I'll never truly understand the bond between a mother and her child.

If that's the case, then they will never understand the bond I have with mine.

I could choose to take all this on board in a negative way, draining at my soul, or I could take it as a lived and learned experience. So instead, I chose to see these as opportunities to raise awareness. Some people are blissfully ignorant without ever knowing it, and I believe ignorance is sometimes simply a result of nurture gone wrong.

Family is not simply about genetics or DNA, it's about the love we have in our hearts and how we choose to share that love.

"Not being biologically related to a child, doesn't make you any less of a parent. Being a real parent isn't in the DNA, it's in the heart"- Motherhood: The Uncut Truth

A friend recently wrote this to me, and just when I needed it:

'… with no disrespect to biological families and mothers, the love you have for your kids is different Sandra, it's beyond unconditional and there is something even more special about the connection you have with them and the love you give them. Even though those children are not biologically yours, and you didn't give birth to them, the fact you can willingly at the drop of a hat welcome them into your home, and into your heart is truly inspiring. It really is love. Unconditional motherly love.'

The love I have for my children ***is*** different. Despite no biological connection to any of my kids, I still choose to accept them, love them wholeheartedly and unconditionally.

I feel their pain and their hurt. When they cry and share yet another sad story, I cry as I wipe their tears and embrace them. When they are happy, I share in their joy.

Like I said already, we very **consciously chose** this parenting pathway. We knew early on our destiny was fostering or adoption. Why would we bring more helpless little lives into the world, when there are literally millions of children around the world in need of a safe, stable and loving home.

I'm not sure what it is for other parents, even those who struggle time and again with fertility and spend thousands and thousands of dollars to create a child that shares a piece of each of their own DNA – Is it something that perhaps makes them feel less than if their children don't possess some part of their genetic makeup? Is it a fear of the type of adult they will become?

Just as we are able to find and nurture the unconditional love of our chosen partner or mate in life, why is it so hard for so many, to the find the same ability to unconditionally love children who are without homes and in need of love?

I know and understand fostering is not for everyone. It's certainly not an easy pathway. We are living proof of that, and we know the struggles of just how hard it can be.

When our fostering journey first began, we were clear about wanting teenagers. They were the ones the system protected the least. They were not small, vulnerable newborn babies. They often self-select their unendorsed placements, couch surfing, and bouncing from hostel, to group home, to foster placement and back again.

Call us crazy (many did), but the youth workers in us both wanted the opportunity to love, nurture and provide what we could to the young people who we saw were continually let down and moved around.

Even the Department initially struggled to understand our desire to foster teens, instead always trying to offer us babies and small children. But we stood our ground.

It wasn't easy. Teenagers can be hard work, anyway right? But teenagers continually let down by a broken system can be next level. There have been PLENTY of "I hate you" moments, slammed bedroom doors, and nasty name calling thrown our way, but I am still to this day, both surprised and saddened by the ability of other 'foster carers,' service providers or any kind of significant other in a young person's life to so easily give up on them.

The anger you witnessed? A lonely cry for help.

Those tears you wiped? An emotional outlet to combat the pain.

The tantrum that was thrown? That's a child with a history of significant trauma you may never truly understand.

Yes, some days are hard, but the good always outweigh the bad. So much laughter, happiness, and joy, so many practical jokes and pranks, family outings, motorbike rides. The good always make the bad days, worth it.

Despite the anger, outbursts and meltdowns, I still always find it in my heart to love them.

We have fought (and still fight) more battles in their defence than any of them will ever realise or know. Behind closed doors, in what seem like endless meetings, none of them know about the continual arguments and debates we have, defending them and advocating for them.

Even when they thought the worst, we always and unconditionally fought for their best.

It takes a long time with each and every teen that enters our home, to build a bond and a level of trust, that shows them we do actually love them. It's a new experience not only for them, but for us too. They have often not experienced the kind of love we offer, so it sometimes confuses them. They have been hurt and moved around so much in their young lives, that they never want to get too attached. Instead it's easier for them to try as much as they can to just push us away.

I have not one regret. The best decision we ever made was fostering. I love being a mum.

I have always been a strong believer in 'everything happens for a reason.' While my growth has been supported by my ancestors, I also believe no matter how sad or devastating or happy a situation is for us, it ultimately has the ability to shape, alter and change us. We may not see or understand what that is immediately, and it may take years to truly realise the why behind something happening, but I believe everything happens for a reason; to serve a greater purpose.

Truth is, I wouldn't change a thing. Every struggle, tear, laugh, memory made has all been worth it for the people we have both become.

We are human, we all make mistakes, but it is not our mistakes that define or limit us, only our fears, and then, only if we give them the power to do so. Every day we wake up, we are given a second chance at life. So, I choose to embrace each and every moment. Learn from past mistakes, heal from the grief and loss, focus on the today, with hope for my tomorrow.

Essentially my ancestors and the love and teachings of both my parents, led me to where I am today. To where I am meant to be.

It led me to pursue youth work. My mother's love and influence on me especially led me to choose this pathway.

It led me to meet and find love with Dave. We share a love and passion for our work, and together we have built our own family.

In a weird way, my life has gone full circle.

I feel as though Dave and I have together created a similar home to the one I grew up in. A home and family of inclusivity, protection, welcoming and unconditional love.

As women, matriarchs who are rising, we all have a story to share. We all have a message inside of us to convey. Many are already out there spreading their messages, and rising to the occasion, lifting and supporting others around them. The rest of us are still simply finding our way out of our (robotically seeming) desensitised, pre-conditioned, and for years beforehand, caged minds and souls, to truly find the power inside of us, and ultimately become the rising matriarch.

And so, the journey of writing this chapter, in this book, is the start of my new beginning, it is me rising to the occasion, as I evolve into a matriarch.

Acknowledging my past, I accept that every challenge I have faced has been for a reason. I have grown. My inner voice has grown. I have now truly come to embrace the strong, fiery woman within myself. For years, I thought I was strong, but upon reflection I now realise how scared and quietly reserved my inner spirit was.

That was me then. This is me now.

The new matriarch.

To those who stood idly by watching as I fell – I dare you to watch me now as I rise.

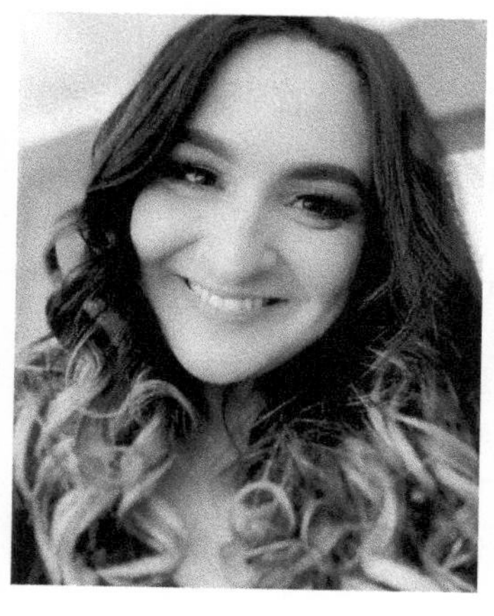

Sandra Erica

Mother | Social Entrepreneur | Author | Speaker | Professional Youth Practitioner & Youth Service Consultant | Fashion (Runway & Photographic) Creative Director & Producer | Qualified & Experienced G&D Educator | Change Maker | Social Justice Advocate

This chapter is my story however I MUST first acknowledge, respect and pay tribute to she, who leads us now. People don't truly know how humble this strong seeming - from the exterior view at least - Matriarch of my own family, my mother Teresa, actually is.

I hold her in such high regard, that I have chosen to dedicate this chapter to her. I hope to one day be just like her - strong, resilient and so incredibly humble. Compassionate, empathetic, understanding and kind. Fierce, loyal and respected.

She has experienced significant pain, heart ache, grief, loss, trauma, stress, anxiety and depression. But her resilience has made her bounce back from many a difficult situation. Because beneath it all, she is a *WARRIOR*, a fighter, a survivor; just like our ancestors who walked before us.

In a small Italian village, at just 2 years of age, she lost her own mother. Never an opportunity to say goodbye. Never knowing the location of her mother's final resting place. My Nonna was very suddenly and heartbreakingly taken away from all of her 5 children at just 29 years of age, after falling ill, never to return home again. It was suspected she may have had a brain tumour. No understanding by her children of what had actually killed her, no funeral for her children to mourn her loss. How does one truly mourn their loss, with their mother's final resting place unknown?

Mum never had a biological mother to grow her up, or show her love, instead she was raised by her strict but incredibly loving and humble father. He re-married and she was then co-raised by a stepmother, who made her life all kinds of hell – however talk to my mum, and even still to this very day she would not dare utter an ill word against her stepmother. Because deep inside her, she is continually filled with forgiveness, compassion and empathy. She always believed and also made me believe, that everyone is unique, individual and some kind of quirky in their own individual way. She taught me to love everyone as they are.

My mother holds close to her so many secrets of others that she never repeats. She is trusted, she has an incredibly big heart and she is one of the most kind-hearted humans I have ***EVER*** known. She's the type of sister you need in your tribe, the one cheering in your corner, and loyally stationing herself at your side, but with access to a loud and inspirational voice when needed - and no matter what, she does not judge, discriminate or turn against you.

I am an unconditionally loving mother, an extremely passionate youth worker and a fighter for important causes I believe in.

I want to change the world, and I believe I will change the world.

I'm a dreamer and a believer. I believe anything is possible.

I want women to stop tearing each other down, to work together and build each other up, nurturing each other's growth, fixing each other's crowns (even when she doesn't see you do it).

I want to defend those who are not there to speak for themselves.

I want to continue to be the voice of those who have been silenced.

Some things I'm most passionate about changing, are; Combatting Racism, Gender Equality, Women's Rights, Family and Domestic Violence, Rates of regional and remote Youth Suicide, Increased access to professionally developed and implemented youth services to regional and remote young people, Raising awareness of the types of parenting and explaining the reality of life for fosters and Challenging others to think outside the box when it comes to DNA, Genetics and Parenting.

I have been incredibly blessed to have worked as a Youth Worker for over 22 years. A vast majority of my career has been place-based, outreach model service delivery, living and working in some of Australia's most remote locations for extended periods of time. I am particularly passionate about the development and sustainability of professional Youth Work practice in Regional and Remote areas.

Following many years of remote Youth Work, I developed a deep passion for raising the awareness of the importance of the professional youth work role in regional and remote locations, working to educate and positively shift mistaken views and mindsets of the youth work role to communities and their elders, and working towards service continuity and sustainability through inclusion of local community people in paid positions and having them afforded the opportunity to complete youth work qualifications.

In 2015, together with my husband Dave, I co-founded Blue Beanie Projects, a not for profit health promotion charity working with 5-25 year olds - aimed at increasing regional children and young people's access to professional, ethical and sustainable youth services; and to increase young people's self-esteem, confidence, resilience, social and emotional wellbeing, health and connection to community.

The charity motto is: The Spirit of Youth - Strong, Resilient, Empowered.

Blue Beanie believe with access to appropriate *professional* services, delivered by suitably qualified and experienced youth workers, they can help reduce the staggering rates of youth suicide in regional and remote locations.

While for the time being, I have chosen to step away from the management side of the organisation, focussing now instead on my writing endeavours, I have chosen to donate ***all profits*** from any sales of my personal copies of this book, to Blue Beanie Projects.

Email: SandraErica@mail.com
Mobile: 0439 983 549
Instagram: @SandraEricaInOz
Facebook: SandraEricaAuthor
LinkedIn: sandra-erica-4a1bab48
Clubhouse: @SandraErica

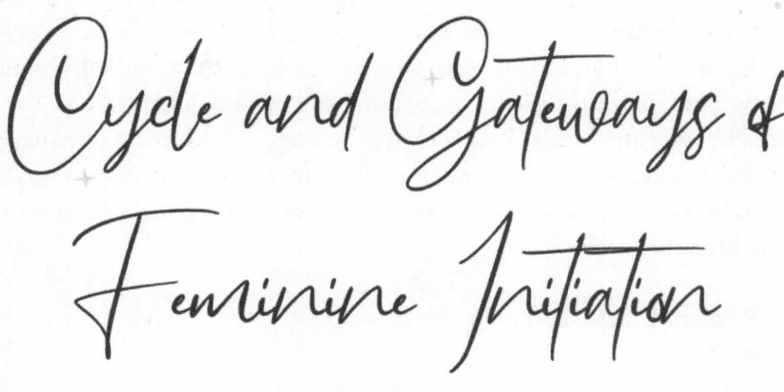

Cycle and Gateways of Feminine Initiation

Sohalia Fitzgerald

In my overall inner landscape at fifty-seven, l can sense that l have definitely landed, and keep landing, deeper into my authentic self. l can feel that l am truer and less wavering in my centre than ever before. The greatest part of my journey has being in the transitional and initiatory space of menopause. l just didn't know the depths of this recalibration and the extent of the cycle of death and rebirth. It has been, and still continues to be, a profound unbecoming and becoming on the physical, mental, emotional, spiritual and soul level. It is my lived experience that as my roots deepen and expand into my true nature, l simultaneously feel the physical roots and connection to this earthly plane loosen and wither.

If l can grow into being, conscious, accepting, and welcoming to this cycle then l believe l can connect even deeper to the beauty of this last adventure.

With every step in our journey as women, there is a death of what was and a birthing of something new. We embrace this so readily with the child to maiden and maiden to mother. Yet this last cycle is often degraded and eroded. rather than seen as the crowning glory of our journey. And l reference the word crown, in relation to the term, 'Crone,' which means crowned one, 'Hag,' which means holy one, and 'Witch,' which means wise one. Those words in the modern world conjure up distorted, ugly and whizzled up images of women; shunned, reviled and cast away from the world of meaning and power .We are here to change that.

So this chapter is a sharing around the flow of one cycle into another.

Menopause is often referred to as 'the change,' even though all phases of the feminine journey are associated with epic changes. l even had a book called MeNoPause, suggesting that there was no need to stop or pause, because with the support of bio-identical hormones you can just keep on keeping on at your usual pace. This feels like the constant message of the modern world. Don't allow space, don't reflect, don't slow down. It's only a physiological process and an annoyance at least, or a devastation to ignore, at most.

As an over-doer already, keeping up my usual pace was the opposite to what my body, emotions and spirit needed. Eight years into this journey and listening to other women's lived experience, this was the very time needed to pause, a LOT. It was a time to take in the internal scenery, as well as, the external surroundings (work, relationships, lifestyle, patterns and habits). Everything was up for review and scrutiny. Space. So often I just needed space; so much fucking space with no one in it except the quiet and beauty of nature. Other times I needed other women, a close friend, sister or mother surrounding me. Sometimes I needed the safe harbour of being held by my beloved, while I clung on to him and my sanity.

Whilst I came to Menopause pretty ignorant to the magnitude of the journey, I arrived into menopause deeply connected to my blood cycle and assumed that this would hold me in good stead, as I entered the next gateway.

I have read how in many traditional cultures, when living in close community, that women's moon (bleeding) cycles were often aligned. I have had the lived experience (as I am sure many of you reading this have), of that happening in houses shared with other women. Because that's what we do; it's one of those, 'we are part of nature things,' a crazy thought in a patriarchal world.

The women bleeding would go into ceremony, rest and move away from daily life in the village. This precious shedding wasn't experienced as shame or mess but as holy blood because it held the potential for giving life. Women were seen in some cultures, as being so powerful that they could not participate in mixed ceremonies.

I once knew an artist who collected her blood in her moon cup and would paint with it. How wonderful and what an act of rebellion.

In my early bleeding days I was lost in the dogma of shame and hiding myself. Sexually if I was on my moon time. I would spray my undies with Charlie perfume (very 70's), and I used tampons which I also learnt were not for me. But at the time, I wanted to plumb up and dam the red river that wanted to remind me of my feminine power and cycle.

Women can be innies or outies just like belly buttons. Innies, like moon cups or tampons, and don't enjoy the wetness or sensation of blood trickling. Outies, as I found myself to be, preferred the flow to flow, as I would get cramps or discomfort in my belly using a tampon.

I am eternally grateful that when in my thirties and life was turbulent and going pear-shaped, (my lesbian phase), I took a deep dive into saving my soul and filling the gaping hole in me that was full of pot and tobacco.

I randomly committed to a year of learning the native American Indian ways. (Yes my teacher had legitimate lineage and permission to teach). She had worked as a journalist and l read one of her articles about their traditional relationship and understanding of women's moon time. It was literally the first time l had ever read that women's blood, my blood, was sacred and that l could create ritual around this monthly event.

As I was a nurse, l had somehow scored an operating theatre towel - green, big and thick material. They were used for patients post-op to keep them warm. They were thick and heavy, but also absorbent for other bodily fluids l won't mention.

The lovely receptionist in our small community hospice team helped me out by cutting, sewing and overlocking the towel into face washer-size pieces of cloth. l would fold them into three to create a make shift pad and pop it into my knickers. Heavy with blood, I would then put them into a watering can full of water. l would watch them sink with the pink and red swirls of my sacred blood as it gently mixed with the water; blood and water dissolving into each other like a caress.

l was in a very paradoxical time in my life, On one level l felt liberated sexually, as l was deeply in love in a relationship with a woman. Intimacy during times of bleeding became an act of revolution, defiance, pleasure and empowerment for me. l reclaimed something very primal and basic to not feel abhorrence towards my blood. All the yuck l had so inherently felt, that was programmed in by what Clarissa Pinkola Estes calls the 'over culture,' left.

All the yuck l felt, handed down by generations of my female lineage, evaporated. It was an incredibly poignant and important point in my journey as a woman. Paradoxically at this time, l was lost in addiction. My world with a partner who was a musician, consisted of gigs, pubs, a lot of binge drinking and binge smoking of tobacco and cannabis … a story for later.

So back to the watering can, which impregnated with the red water, l would use to water the plants. My life-giving sacred blood mixed with life-giving water. l was able to gift real and meaningful nourishment to the plant world and the earth. On reflection, l realise now how this ritual or practice gave me something life-affirming and supportive to do with my blood as l had chosen to not bring children through my body this life time - yet another story.

It brought meaning, purpose, happiness and peace to me that l was able to use my blood to nurture and feed living things. It also brought me a powerful ritual every month, even though at the time, it felt so ordinary and simple.

Years later, after more adventures and exploration, l married a magnificent human. l initiated him into my sacred monthly blood practice and would regularly ring him at work, happily announcing that my moon time had arrived and how much joy I felt. I loved that he would water the plants and not be freaked out by my now, soaked and rinsed blood cloths, popping them into the wash and hanging them on the line. These were good days.

So fast-track a decade or so later and you can probably imagine that I was not keen on my moon time EVER stopping. Given the option, I would have happily bled every twenty-one days for the rest of my life. I used this time as a reset, as a cleanse and as a lived connection to mother nature and a bigger, more ancient, feminine wisdom. So with that mindset firmly entrenched, I didn't investigate or show any interest in what I may experience in the CHANGE called Menopause.

I simply rested in the inertia, and relied on the indoctrination of my time; that of TV, movies [bad movies], magazines, biological facts and other limited resources.

So my understanding of what was to come focused around being moody, (same program assigned to menstruation), my yoni would dry up, my libido would be finished, there would be hot flushes and I would become a rectangular shape, losing my feminine curves. Plus, I would resort to having short, short hair (nothing wrong with that). The biggest story though, was that I would become invisible, and don the mask of the sweet grey-haired, not so boisterous, soft-nanna type. Not one of those hag like creatures depicted in fairy tales.

I knew that women's cycles often become erratic, with starts and stops. There could be break through bleeding mid cycle or the dreaded flood of blood.

I loved my cycle so much that I started an unconscious prayer.

I often spoke to Paul, to women friends, my mother and my sisters, that my heartfelt wish was to not be tortured with my cycle stopping, and then in the midst of my grieving, have it return. Like a game of cat and mouse. When the time came, my wish was it would stop and never return. And it did exactly that in June 2013. My moon time never returned and another story began.

In the beginning there were the warm flushes and I was ok with that, very doable, not pleasant but ok.

Over the years my connection to spirit and the beginnings of self -love had grown. This came to be mainly through engaging in shamanic practices, skilled counselling and conscious dance. Not so oddly, my alcohol and substance intake lessened.

However, often in the times that I would indulge, it is fair to say I would get my drinking and smoking booties well on. The cleaner I got, the more awake and alive I felt - in a good good way.

According to the World Health Organisation, I read that the safe limit for women's consumption of alcohol is 125mls; a dismal quarter of a glass (Why bother?) Even with restraint l found that to be, 1) very unappealing, and 2) very unsatisfying. So alcohol left my world. At the time l failed to link these habits with having been a form of me self-medicating a life long sympathetic dominant and traumatised nervous system. l failed to understand that l had relied on these since my twenties to calm, to cope, and for emotional and mental pain relief.

So l came into the full force of menopause cold turkey and raw, and didn't have an inkling of what was about to happen

l remember reading somewhere that there are sixty-six symptoms associated with menopause.

The most debilitating for me long term, was having no restorative sleep for four years. l was not aware that l slept lightly, except that each morning l woke up depleted. In a nostalgic moment, l tried a friend's cannabis brownie and woke up the next day feeling deeply rested. It was a big 'ah ha' moment as l realised l had adjusted to sleep deprivation being my norm.

l was easily triggered into distress, overwhelm, anger, and irritability. Fight, flee and freeze were constant responses to seemingly trivial and minor triggers. l would walk around the house not knowing what to do or what l was meant to do. Doing dishes and simple tasks were insurmountable, leading to tears and panic.

The warm flushes became the karmic fires of hell. They left me covered in a constant sheen of moisture day and night, with an uncomfortable sticky sensation. I would kick off the bedclothes to then become clammy and cold, then haul them back on. I was not able to touch my partner , or be touched, as it would trigger another round of flushing, as would rolling over in bed.

Each morning, l roused with a sweat and a sensation of dread or impending doom, that started in my lower belly, and like a wave washed into my throat and into the front of my skull. Often there was no story, just the sensation of overwhelm and defeat even before my feet touched the floor. The eczema, l had pre-adolescence, returned. I experienced reflux, weight gain and my hair thinned. Now l understood why short hair was a thing. Not only practical but desirable, as my hair lacked body, thickness and health. l took a radical approach having grown up with short hair and got dreads instead. (Still have them and love them!)

My memory was shot to pieces. Old trauma and wounds long thought to be healed arose like an army of vicious ghosts, haunting me and creating distress in my relationships and family dynamics. l was sick all the time, like l had never been, catching every cold and virus. l went down with no resilience just wanting to hide beneath the covers. But hiding in bed did not help, it only heightened the isolation and feeling of drowning. l knew exercise and meditation would help but I was too exhausted; too exhausted and fried to meditate and I felt like a caged animal pacing restlessly looking for a way out.

As the life I knew crumbled, I took to my situation like a detective, as desperation was sweeping away everything that anchored me. I read books on the gut, hormones, took notes and filled journals, I saw naturopaths, healers, and therapists for body, mind and soul. That's when I came to see and understand the level of deep anxiety and trauma in my system. I read particularly about the vagus nerve and the nervous system, bringing compassion and understanding to these uncharted waters.

I created my own symptom score sheet, with fifteen major symptoms, so I could score the severity (0-5) and track myself. With my memory shot, I was unreliable, life was unreliable and I continued to ask myself, 'what if this was it for me?' Most of what I tried worked for my friends going through menopause, but not me, Even CBD oil , which I thought would be the holy grail, failed me. Two drops a night and increase by two until you slept. I got to twelve drops and called it quits.

I finally decided to explore bio-identical hormones; not the synthetic, chemical kind, but the ones that match what a woman's body produces. After my body failed to absorb the hormone cream, I went on to unfortunately have weird and extreme reactions to the troche (lozenger) and pessary. So another avenue for relief and support was closed.

Every path I traversed led to either no effect or a side effect. So much was collapsing; my gut, my nervous system, my mental health and all my physical resilience. I touched places where I wanted out of this body and this world.

But as they say in the classics, 'my breakdown was my break through.'

I had been collecting so many books, I finally noticed a book that had sat on my shelf for a good year or so. Previously daunted by its encyclopedial size, I started to read and discovered information that was helpful on every level. (The Wisdom of Menopause by Dr. Christiane Northrup).

I learnt that my brain was being completely rewired so that I would literally not be the same person once everything recallibrated .

I learnt that the level of hormones flooding my system was akin to adolescence, no real surprises there, in terms of the extreme emotional states I was experiencing.

I learnt that the memory centres of my brain were being flooded by hormones, causing old memories, some known and some long forgotten, to be re-activated. I wasn't looking for trouble, I wasn't consciously creating pain for myself, this was physiologically happening to me.

The hormones designed to keep the peace, to be the diplomat or overlook aspects in life which didn't feel ok, were leaving. And the bug eyes of unavoidable seeing and truth were taking its place.

But on a deeper level, what was taking up residence was the real me; the woman, no longer by design, manipulated by a monthly hormonal soup. And what I was experiencing was a huge purging, amplified because I came to this unprepared and because I had given the process no priority or space to unfold. The anxiety and traumatised nervous system that had always being there, was now demanding my attention, my love, my presence and space to move. Everything was unfiltered, and no longer sedated, and these parts of me refused to sit on the side lines any longer .

Something shifted and I saw the power in the pain. I saw the movement towards something arriving; a birthing of myself. At first, that knowing was a tiny speck of dust, but it was a lifeline that slowly grew resilience, courage, belief and trust.

This journey was way bigger, way more encompassing and was leading me to discover, define and embody the REAL, fully-alive me.

I read The Body Keeps The Score by Bessel Van Der Kolk and life brought me a Somatic Experiencing therapist in the shape of a trusted friend doing the training, One of the most supportive things he shared was a sense he had that menopausal women were, at times, almost therapy resistant in their journey. They seek help, and want help. They are committed to the process. They gain insight and even experience a shift, but then, like the half finished jigsaw puzzle on the table, someone [in this case menopause] comes in and swipes all the pieces on the floor and you start again. Back to the drawing board, again and again. This reflection brought acceptance and kindness to myself, and the journey.

Coffee left, gluten left, histamine-rich foods left. Thanks to another wise friend's advice, when I got swallowed by the overwhelm, she would say the following. Find three to five seconds of 'no thoughts' which was a breath, [I could do that]. Then find three things in the present moment that I could be grateful for. Once I found three, I could often find more and it broke the back of many a black, sticky sink-hole.

I have been told that there is a correlation with increased admission rates into psychiatric care and severe menopausal symptoms.

I wonder about the rate of menopausal women being prescribed anti-depressants.

I also wonder about the increase of alcohol consumption to manage symptoms, such as anxiety and sleep disturbance during menopause.

Biofeedback taught me how to calm my system and tap into tools to activate my parasympathetic nervous system (moving out of the sympathetic, fight, flight, freeze).

Neurofeedback found my unsupportive unconscious default wiring, which explained much of how I had responded and was responding to life. I sat week after week with electrodes on my head, mapping out a new healthier default pathway. It also, coincidently and weirdly, appeared to activate a dream, which felt at the time to be a deep remembering of a horrific trauma. What unfolded over a ten month period is nothing short of magic, but again a story for another time …

What I learnt at the core was I hadn't met myself in this place of transition. So I had to be brought kicking screaming on my knees, before I gave it, and all of me, my full attention. Approaching this journey as transactional or purely physical was so short sighted.

Because of its impact in scuttling life as I knew it, I also treated it and my body as the enemy and not the teacher and healer it has become. This journey is absolutely one of change with losses (what isn't in all our cycles?) But ultimately, it can consciously be about arriving into a place of power, centredness, vibrancy and visibility. Many women across the world are living in a time where we are more educated than the centuries preceding. Many of us are more financially independent than before. The bonds of religious dogma and restrictions [for many] have been lifted or eased compared to a century ago. According to Dr. Christiane Northrup, menopausal women make up the largest percentage of the world population. I didn't know that, and to me, that signals a whole lot of power and capacity to drive change. I believe we can be inspiring and capable game-changers and way-seers in this world. Free from the other aspects of the feminine journey, we can bring our knowledge, our wisdom and creativity to lead and find solutions for humanity (in partnership with our brothers). So lets get visible, shine our light and create a map for our younger sisters to follow with self-love and empowerment at the heart of the journey

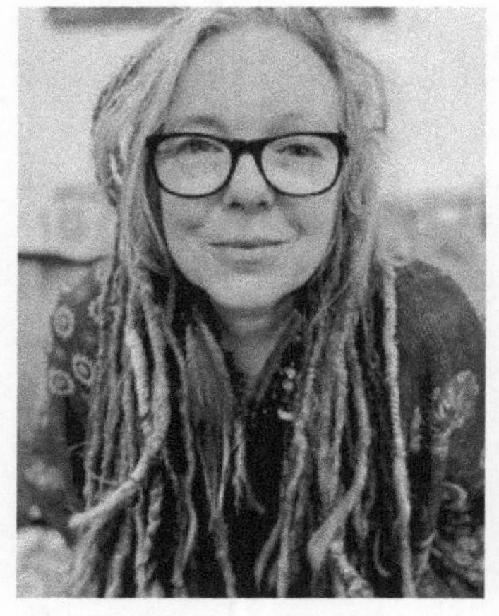

Sohalia Fitzgerald

I am a woman celebrating the last half of my life and l bring consciousness and a welcoming to this knowing.

Living fully and moving towards death with the intention that noTHING will have a hold or tether me to the life being left behind. The only thread will be love and that will be the vehicle to support and propel me into flight (with her arms wide open).

l arrived in a time when TV was new and seen as a wonder and source of all things good. The deep programming through this medium, magazines and the over culture around being a girl and a woman ran deep. Even to this day it requires ever-vigilant enquiry, recognition, awareness and constant shedding.

At 14 years of age l was hit at high speed by a car on the way to school; a near-death experience and an event that shaped much of my life.

As a dancer from 5 to 13 years of age, this door slammed shut after the accident.

But dance found its way in clubs, pubs, raves and then in the emergence of the conscious dance movement. This started in the late 90's . In dance, l touched my beauty. It is my place to safely explore and release. A place to express and discover more and more layers. Layers for shedding, layers for awakening, and layers for celebrating. 5 Rythms, Biodanza, Wu Tao, Open floor and especially Ritual Trance Dance.

The accident brought many gifts and led firstly to a career working with children. From then l mid-wifed at the other end of the spectrum and had 24 years of palliative nursing in hospice and the community. A reflexologist, l specialised in maternity and cancer support for some years. Currently l work part-time as a continence Nurse Advisor. A fitting career as the accident left me with stress incontinence from the age for 14.

Shamanic ritual and earth-based practices have been my tools, providing me with guidance, healing and connection to myself and the earth.

l facilitate Ritual Trance Dance, a contemporary dance ritual created in the 1980's. It incorporates conscious intention, breath of fire, blindfolded dance / movement and integration. It provides a safe place for deep self-enquiry, exploration, and freedom to move, as no one is watching. Participants are able to access visionary states and the ritual invites an expanded embodied state of consciousness.

My home is an altar and I create with a wild turbulence, saying yes to so many expressions. Writing, art, crochet, sound and dance are all in the mix. My life is big, messy and delightful. I revel in loving others, and being a safe haven for friends in troubled waters (another gift of a difficult life path).

I have a yearning to grow and continue stretching myself until my last breath.

I have loved, being loved and experienced more beauty and love than that 14 year old girl ever knew was possible. I am ordinary and special just like YOU.

www.sohaliapoppins.com
Facebook: dancegroundaustralia

Printed in Australia
AUHW020925040521
345040AU00003B/3

9 780645 135350